PRAISE FOR *WORKING OUT SUCKS!*

"I get it. Working out is hard. But here's another truth: exercise is the only way to improve your health, elevate your mood, increase your energy, prevent illness and injuries, and enhance the overall quality of your life. That's no BS, and neither is *Working Out Sucks!*—so grab a copy and get on track to getting healthy."

—Tony Horton, creator of P90X workout program and author of *Bring It!*

"With its full-prescription 21-day plan, *Working Out Sucks!* presents a 'kick in the pants' approach to unlocking your potential—a longer, healthier ever after."

—Andrea Metcalf, fitness trainer and author of *Naked Fitness*

"*Working Out Sucks!* provides great tips for helping you get on a path towards healthier living. Take the first step and pick up this book—the time to change your future is NOW!"

—Tara Costa, season 7 finalist on *The Biggest Loser*, and founder of Inspire Change Foundation

"This is an important book. It is the first fitness book I know of that is written for those of us who don't enjoy exercising. As such, it's the first, and perhaps the only, fitness book that accepts the fact that most people, most of the time believe that 'working out sucks.' Read on!"

—John McCarthy, Executive Director of the International Health Sports Racquet Club Association (IHRSA) from 1981–2006

WORKING OUT SUCKS!

WORKING OUT
SUCKS!
(and why it doesn't have to)

THE ONLY 21-DAY KICK-START PLAN
FOR TOTAL HEALTH AND FITNESS
YOU'LL EVER NEED

CHUCK RUNYON

with Brian Zehetner, MS, RD, CSSD, CSCS
and Rebecca A. DeRossett, MSW, LICSW

Da Capo
LIFE
LONG

A Member of the Perseus Books Group

Copyright © 2012 by Anytime Fitness, LLC

Library of Congress Cataloging-in-Publication Data is available for this book.

ISBN 978-0-7382-1569-3
ISBN 978-0-7382-1573-0 (e-Book)

First Da Capo Press edition 2012

Published by Da Capo Press
A Member of the Perseus Books Group
www.dacapopress.com

Book design by Jane Raese
Set in 10-point Linoletter

Editorial production by Marrathon Production Services. www.marrathon.net

Note: The information in this book is true and complete to the best of our knowledge. This book is intended only as an informative guide for those wishing to know more about health issues. In no way is this book intended to replace, countermand, or conflict with the advice given to you by your own physician. The ultimate decision concerning care should be made between you and your doctor. We strongly recommend you follow his or her advice. Information in this book is general and is offered with no guarantees on the part of the authors or Da Capo Press. The authors and publisher disclaim all liability in connection with the use of this book.

Many of the designations used by manufacturers and sellers to distinguish their products are claimed as trademarks. Where those designations appear in this book and Da Capo Press was aware of a trademark claim, the designations have been printed in initial capital letters.

Da Capo Press books are available at special discounts for bulk purchases in the U.S. by corporations, institutions, and other organizations. For more information, please contact the Special Markets Department at the Perseus Books Group, 2300 Chestnut Street, Suite 200, Philadelphia, PA, 19103, or call (800) 810-4145, ext. 5000, or e-mail special.markets@perseusbooks.com.

10 9 8 7 6 5 4 3 2

*To anyone who struggles with motivation
to improve their life, don't give up.*

*You're worth every bead of sweat.

*And to all those who bleed purple—
we have inspired many,
but our work is not done.*

BOOK PROFITS DON'T SUCK
(But We're Giving Them Away)

I hope this book inspires you in new and unexpected ways. And I'd like you to know that as part of our motivation in writing it, we've decided to give away 100 percent of the net proceeds to an incredibly inspiring organization called Limbs for Life.

Limbs for Life is a global nonprofit organization that provides fully functional prosthetic care for individuals who can't otherwise afford it. After twenty years of listening to flimsy excuses from able-bodied people, it's refreshing to meet individuals who, despite everyday struggles consider it a privilege (rather than an annoyance) to be physically active.

Yes, working out sucks . . . but you shouldn't have to lose a limb to appreciate the ones you have. Take a lesson from the people who work at Limbs for Life, and the amputees they serve: They don't just aspire to walk again; they want to run!

To learn more, visit www.limbsforlife.org.

—Chuck Runyon, September 2011

CONTENTS

PART 1: WORKING OUT SUCKS, BUT . . .

PART 4: FITNESS SUCKS TOO, BUT . . .

PART 1

WORKING OUT SUCKS, BUT . . .

CHUCK RUNYON

Working out sucks. There, I said it. I'm the CEO and co-founder of the largest co-ed fitness franchise on the planet, and I'm looking you straight in the eye and telling you: Working out sucks.

Why would I say something that might hurt my business? Because I'm tired of seeing marketing images of lean, glistening, uber-muscled "exertrons" flashing their bleachy white smiles as they work their asses into chiseled granite. You and I know the truth: For the average bear, working out is a chore whose popularity ranks somewhere behind window washing, gutter cleaning and dog poop scooping.

Actually, when it comes to health and wellness, we live in a unique, best-of-times/worst-of-times era. If you're a committed fitness enthusiast, you're well served by over thirty thousand commercial fitness centers in the United States—including YMCAs; women-only clubs; amenity-rich multi-purpose centers; niche operations that focus on Pilates, yoga, or personal training; cheap clubs; expensive clubs; single-gender clubs; and 24/7 clubs. If you include the offerings in hotels, apartment buildings, high schools, and colleges, as well as employer-based facilities, home gyms, children's fitness franchises, stroller fitness for stay-at-home moms, businesses that focus on weight loss and nutrition, smartphone apps, infomercial products, and the tens of thousands of certified personal trainers—there's definitely an affordable fitness option to suit everyone.

But for most people who want to be healthy, these are the worst of times. Health-club options abound, but a tater tot is still way more accessible than a treadmill. A simple stop at the gas station is a full-court sensory assault of fresh bakery smells wafting amid aisles of candy bars and chips. Within minutes of work or home, dozens of fast-food brands offer cheap meals loaded with hundreds (if not thousands) of calories wrapped in overdoses of sodium and sugar. Restaurants compete in a portion-size nuclear arms race. And thanks to smartphone technology, you can now order a movie, get a large pizza with cheese-jammed crust, download a newspaper, walk your avatar dog, and talk to your friends and family without exercising anything more than your thumbs. Plus, we're just busier now. Texts, instant messaging, and social media have crept into every waking hour. And when you add the pressures of raising kids in a sports-obsessed, parents-need-to-be-involved-in-everything culture, we have little time or energy left for exercise.

Technology gives us the illusion of accomplishing more by allowing us to physically accomplish virtually nothing.

That's the genesis of this book: to help the busy ones who hate working out. This is for the people who join a club and go only during the New Year's resolution crunch. The people who get an elliptical machine for Christmas and use it to hang their clothes. The people who get winded walking up a flight of stairs. Anyone who's scared, intimidated, uneducated, unmotivated, or just plain lazy. Or who lacks the genetic blessings to be lean, fit, or coordinated. (I'll be the first to sympathize with those of you born with the "fat gene." I don't care what those meathead trainers say; many people are born with almost no chance to be a hard body with single-digit body fat and six-pack abs.)

But this book isn't about fitting into a teeny bikini or having a tree-trunk neck. It's about living an outrageously fun and fully engaged life—to be in a position where your physical condition makes your life better, instead of limiting it. In short, it's about being as good as your body was born to be.

What makes me an expert? Am I an experienced fitness trainer? Do I hold a doctorate degree in nutrition? No. But I've been a personal witness to human discipline, motivation, and procrastination in the fitness industry in every region of the country. At the age of twenty, I started my career as a part-time membership salesperson at a fitness club while I attended the local college. Within a few months, I was having a blast working in the club and making a better income than most guys my age. When I was twenty-one, two friends and I started a marketing company that traveled the country and helped club owners generate new memberships. For the next six years, I spent nine to ten months working in different fitness centers around the United States and generating thousands of new memberships. This type of travel—and constantly opening a "new business" (a new membership campaign) every two months in a different city—was perfect training to become an entrepreneur. I had to be resourceful, creative, driven, flexible, and responsive while getting along with people of all ages, shapes, genders, races, religions, and incomes.

Over the last twenty-three years, I've witnessed many new offerings that encourage people to commit to a healthier lifestyle. From StairMaster equipment to water aerobics to thirty-minute circuit training to pole dancing—the barrage of new equipment and cleverly branded workout programs by bulging-biceped gurus will never stop. But motivation doesn't start in the health club; it starts in the mind. And that's where I come in.

In my career, I've probably heard more lazy excuses and flat-out lies than anyone else on the planet. But it's funny, even as the fitness industry has changed, the excuses haven't. Twenty years ago, the three most common reasons for not joining a club were these:

1. "I don't have the time."
2. "I can't afford it."
3. "I can't commit."

These are still the three most popular excuses today.

But this book isn't here to convince you to join a club. Really, it's not. Obviously, if you do decide to go that route, I hope you choose Anytime Fitness. But I just want you to be active. To be healthier. To make your world and our world a better place.

The fact is, I don't think of this as a book. It's a deprogramming effort. Along with fat, salt, and sugar, we're all filled with tons of misinformation—and we've treated this issue with kid gloves for too long. I want *Working Out Sucks* to shock you into recognition, hit you on an emotional level, and dispel the biggest health myths you've been fed over the years. I'm not going to fill this book with gloom-and-doom statistics, clinical explanations, and arcane scientific studies. Instead, you'll find a practical 21-day program for getting on the path to change, you'll read success stories from people who've done what you want to do, and you'll be challenged to make this the last health and fitness book you'll ever buy.

If this effort succeeds, you'll go from wanting to *be* healthy to wanting to *get* healthy—and you'll get off your bulbous rump to do something about it. After I slap you upside your head with a supersized dose of motivation (my specialty), Rebecca DeRossett, MSW, LICSW, a marriage, family and behavior-change therapist in Stillwater, Minnesota, will address the unique emotional issues associated with health and wellness. (Health is so often associated with the body, but the real key to success is using the brain to unlock motivation and overcome fear.) Then, Brian Zehetner, MS, RD, CSSD, CSCS, a registered dietitian and a conditioning specialist in Woodbury, Minnesota, will provide a commonsense approach that takes the mystery and intimidation out of fitness and nutrition. I've collaborated with experts because, like you, I also seek outside help to reach my personal fitness and nutrition goals.

So this is it. The journey starts here. If you don't mind a get-real approach to health, then turn the page and begin to treat your life—your full emotional, spiritual, soulful and physical life—seriously. If that doesn't sound good, or you're too sensitive or easily offended, then put this book down, take out your smartphone, and click on the "order a pizza" app.

It's your choice.

FIFTY-FIFTY

"Your son has a fifty-fifty chance of surviving this surgery."

Those were the words heard by my parents in January 1982. My older brother, Steve, was facing heart transplant surgery at the age of seventeen. It's sad to think of any teenager in this situation, but in my brother's case, he could be considered lucky. He was born with a tiny hole in his heart, a condition that prevented the heart from keeping up with his body's circulatory demands—especially during strenuous activities. Shortly after he was born, the doctors didn't think he would live past the age of five.

But Steve had irrepressible resolve, some inexplicable good fortune, and the care of brilliant personnel along the way. Although he was three-and-a-half years older than I was, he was physically weaker. He wasn't strong, and his endurance would be taxed fairly quickly in any athletic event. His condition prevented him from participating in organized sports, but it didn't stop him from playing neighborhood games with his sister, brothers, and friends.

My brother was compassionate toward other kids and patients with physical limitations, and he shunned pity. If he took his shirt off, you could see two massive scars on his chest. One long scar ran down the center of his chest. The other ran horizontally from the front of his ribs and around the side of his body. The scars looked like two sets of railroad tracks on a very skinny body—evidence of two previous open-heart surgeries. After a while, Steve learned to take his shirt off and enjoy life without being self-conscious—despite the constant questions, teasing, and staring.

Steve enjoyed swimming, being outdoors, hiking, and playing football with his younger brother in the park near our home. He would get annoyed at himself for running out of breath and slowing down the games. But after he caught his wind, he'd go right back to them. Steve was robbed of the ability to play without limitations. He had to think twice about every physical action, and it must have been difficult to always be the last kid picked in most games. (Although when I was captain, I always picked him first.)

As Steve got older, his heart began to wear out. The defective organ could not circulate blood effectively, his extremities often grew cold, and his breathing during any strenuous activity—even for a short time—became almost immediately labored. As his situation deteriorated, the medical experts determined that my brother's heart was bound to give out. A heart transplant was the only way to keep him alive.

That brings us back to the fifty-fifty conversation. Can you imagine a coin flip determining your life—or a one-in-two chance of ever seeing your son, daughter, brother, or sister again? That morning in the hospital, just hours before surgery, our family spent our last moments with my brother. What do you say in this situation? Steve had spent countless nights in the hospital and had become accustomed to the heightened emotions. While we cried and hugged each other, he artfully injected humor into conversations, defused the gloom, and refused to succumb to self-pity. We all did our best to be optimistic, to fool ourselves into knowing for certain that we would see him alive later that day. We hoped and prayed, but we didn't know which side of the coin Steve would get.

My brother died on the operating table, surrounded by a brilliant medical team that did everything they could to save him. Although I've summarized his story in a few hundred words, my brother's death has left a void that is still felt thirty years later by me, my younger brother, my older sister, and my mom and dad. Although Steve was the one born with a hole in his heart, he left a hole in ours. But here's the question: Was my brother lucky or unlucky? If you ask the doctors, they'll say he was lucky. Remember, they didn't predict that he would live past the age of five. But he was fortunate enough to experience almost eighteen years of life. My brother would have agreed with them.

Working out sucks . . . but your excuses suck more. Do your arms and legs work? Does your heart beat? Although few of us were born with the physical gifts to be a professional athlete, most of us were born with a silver spoon in our DNA. Mentally and physically, we have nothing holding us back. The challenges we face are the TV remote, the recliner chair, and an endless barrage of mindless sitcoms. During the final days of my brother's life, he badly wanted to swim before his final surgery. The doctors wouldn't allow it at first, but my parents coaxed them into letting Steve take one more swim. In the pool, he was happy. He felt normal and light, and the water rejuvenated his spirits. All he wanted to do was something you or I can do every day without having to ask for a doctor's permission. Steve wanted to be active. How about you? Unless you were born with a serious malfunction, you have no excuse. You are luckier than you think—even if you were born into a fat family. Get off your ass, quit feeling sorry for yourself, and start living.

THE MAGIC PILL

Right now, in laboratories across the country, some really smart people are working to create a "skinny pill" that will replace the need to exercise. Can you imagine how rich someone would be if he or she could find a way to make us all healthy just by taking a pill?

Still, I hope none of you are holding out for it. Remember Olestra? It was a fat substitute that added no fat, calories, or cholesterol to products, and it had been used in the preparation of traditionally high-fat foods. Everyone was excited at the thought of eating endless potato chips, french fries, and other junk food with no consequences—except for a few side effects, like, um . . . diarrhea. (Not surprisingly, Olestra didn't last long. Consumers wouldn't trade eating a bag of Olestra chips for six trips to the bathroom.)

There's no denying that we live in a pill-obsessed society. And don't get me wrong: I'm not trivializing the necessity of pills or their effectiveness in helping people who have serious conditions. But I've also seen the power of exercise as medicine, and clinical evidence supports the idea that regular exercise lifts mood, increases happiness, decreases stress, and boosts confidence and self-worth.

How we feel about ourselves physically is undeniably important, and this personal appraisal critically influences our conscious choices and subconscious actions every day. Consider this scenario: What if everyone were simply healthier? What if an entire community of individuals experienced a prolonged boost in self-esteem? People with healthy self-esteem get better grades, commit fewer crimes, are less prone to addictions, and have a higher degree of social confidence.[1] And studies have shown that people with high self-esteem report being happier, healthier, and wealthier — and list more close relationships with friends and family members than do people with low self-esteem.

Look at this from another perspective. Listed below is a rap sheet on some of the challenging societal issues that cause pain, conflict, and societal decay:

Crime
Teen pregnancy
Bullying
Sex abuse
Sex addiction
Alcoholism
Drug abuse
Domestic violence
Poor student performance and test scores
Depression
Racism/discrimination

What do all of these issues have in common? In many cases, they originate from low self-esteem. Or, if there's a biological or neurological vulnerability (which has been linked to alcoholism and obesity), psychological deficiencies may develop secondarily. Either way, it's safe to presume that when you look at this list, low self-esteem is both a cause and a result—a vicious circle if there ever was one. So, what happens as an entire generation becomes unhealthier? Considering the list of issues above, how does that manifest into poor decisions or overall societal decay?

Self-esteem is the likeliest candidate for a social vaccine, something that empowers us to live responsibly and that inoculates us against the lures of crime, violence, substance abuse, teen pregnancy, child abuse, chronic welfare dependency, and educational failure. The lack of self-esteem is central to most personal and social ills plaguing our state and nation.

—CALIFORNIA TASK FORCE TO PROMOTE SELF-ESTEEM
AND PERSONAL AND SOCIAL RESPONSIBILITY

Am I suggesting that low self-esteem (being emotionally unhealthy) coupled with being physically unhealthy is one of the primary issues affecting our society? Yes. Am I also suggesting that for many people, regular physical exercise may be the magic pill that could make an individual—and a society—a healthier and better place to live in? Ditto.

Working out sucks . . . but having a low self-worth sucks more. Obsessing about pills will only keep you stuck in your rut, waiting for some elusive future while you get fatter and sicker. Think of exercise as medicine—because it is. Plus, it's less expensive than most things you buy at the pharmacy. (And it doesn't cause diarrhea.)

MUGGING YOURSELF

You're walking down the street when some hoodlums approach and give you a choice: "Your money or your life?" You think about it for a bit. Hmmm . . . I have quite a bit of cash on me. How much am I worth?

Sounds crazy, right? In reality, you wouldn't hesitate to give them your money. But when it comes to fitness, why do so many people list money as one of their top reasons for not getting started?

Over the last twenty years, one of the most common I-can't-join-a-gym excuses is "it's too expensive" or "I can't afford it." That's a flimsy lie, and you know it. In today's culture of hyperconsumerism, spending money is our country's most popular sport. The word *thrifty* only exists in the rental car business and the Boy Scouts' honor code.[1]

The average American spends more money in one month of automobile expenses than he or she does on one year of personal fitness-related expenses. That's a lot of chubby people riding around in nice cars!

But you don't have to save or spend money; you simply have to reevaluate what's important to you. Over the years, I've asked thousands of people to rank their most important priorities in life. The top four answers are religion, family, work, and health. This is further supported by a 2010 Barna Group survey that listed Americans' top priorities as (in order of importance)"family, health, wealth, and faith." So most of us rate health as our life's second-highest priority— yet we spend nothing on it. Why?

Let's look at consumer-spending breakdown prepared by the federal government in 2009 (U.S. Department of Labor, "Consumer Expenditures," April 2009):

U.S. CONSUMER UNIT EXPENDITURES (ANNUAL)
PER HOUSEHOLD

Housing:	$16,920
Transportation:	$8,758
Food:	$6,133
Insurance/pensions:	$5,336
Health care:	$2,853
Entertainment:	$2,698
Apparel and services:	$1,881
Cash contributions:	$1,821
Education:	$945
Miscellaneous:	$808
Personal care:	$588
Alcoholic beverages:	$457
Tobacco:	$323
Reading:	$118
TOTAL:	$49,639

If you divide $49,639 by 365 days in a year, you find it takes the average American $136 a day to exist. Now, consider that an average health club membership is $39 a month, which is $1.30 a day. That's less than 1 percent of your monthly budget—and remember, you ranked health and fitness as your second-highest life priority. Don't you find it interesting that you (and many others) are not dedicating anything to your second-highest priority, and to take action, all you have to do is invest less than 1 percent of your monthly budget?

Working out sucks . . . but using a lack of money as an excuse for staying lethargic, out of shape, and depressed sucks more. You're worth more than a green piece of paper with the face of a president on it. Don't rob yourself of the ability to look better, feel better, play with your kids, and not be out of breath when you take the stairs.

ONE LOUSY PERCENT

Speaking of 1 percent, what's something that every man, woman, and child on this planet has in common—something we all share, regardless of country, gender, age, income level, or astrological sign?

Time.

We all get twenty-four hours in a day. There's no upper, lower, or middle class for time. No time tax that takes hours away from the rich and gives them to the poor. No time inheritance that we can pass along to our grandkids. I can't exchange seven hours of American time for 12.5 hours of Australian time. We are not born with a time gene that gives us more or less time. And we can't pay a personal trainer for more time. Time is unemotional, indiscriminating, and undeterred. It doesn't matter if you live in Malaysia, Malta, or Mexico; you get only twenty-four hours in a day.

It may seem as if we're all busier than ever. But remember, our grandparents had the same amount of time, and our future generations will, too. Time doesn't mind being used, and it doesn't care if you waste it. Time cannot be stopped or paused like TiVo. It just keeps ticking with the maddening, never-ending pursuit of a serial killer in a low-budget horror film.

Time has become our most valued currency, and how we spend it defines us. For the last twenty years, one of the biggest objections to working out is "I don't have the time." Let's look at this from a logical and emotional perspective.

I already mentioned that health is the second-highest priority for most people (after family). We did a financial analysis of health; now let's do a time analysis. Take one week: There are 60 minutes in an hour, 24 hours in a day, and 7 days in a week. That gives you 10,080 minutes every week to spend or waste. If you're a fitness enthusiast or training for a serious athletic event, you may need 60 to 90 minutes of vigorous exercise each day. But if you're the average person who hates working out, all you need to invest is 90 to 120 minutes a week.

That's about 1 percent of your overall week dedicated to the second-highest priority in your life. I repeat: 1 percent.

I understand you're busy. I know you need your sleep. You should devote time to family or school, or maybe you're working two jobs. But isn't spending 1 lousy percent of your week worth less stress, more energy, looking better, feeling better, and simply being healthier? Would you ever consider devoting only 1 percent of your week to your family? Your college work? Your job?

No? Then why would you sacrifice your health? Is it because you really don't have the time, or because it's hard?

Working out sucks . . . but wasting time sucks more. In an era with 24/7 fitness clubs that even have TVs on their machines, is time really an excuse anymore? Combine family time with a strenuous walk. Make yourself exercise in the morning. Whatever it takes. It's 1 percent of your week, for crying out loud. Quit whining and start doing!

"AS LONG AS IT'S HEALTHY"

The preceding is a common response uttered by expectant parents when they are asked the question "Are you hoping for a boy or girl?" But what happens after we're blessed with a healthy baby? Do we keep that child strong and fit, or do we begin feeding it a toxic diet of fat, sodium, sugar, and processed foods?

Does a parent's unconditional love come with conditions?
Because it appears that we'll do anything for our kids—
except exercise or eat healthy for them!

Too often, it's the latter. And if that sounds like a paradox, think about all the inherent contradictions in today's parenting:

- We preach the value of education and instilling positive habits in our children, yet we provide virtually no understanding of the food they eat, nor do we encourage healthy habits and regular physical activity.
- We challenge our kids in the hope that accomplishment breeds self-confidence, and we understand that healthy self-esteem is critical to living a more fulfilling life. Yet, having a poor body image siphons any confidence and self-esteem that we build.

- We protect our kids from all kinds of threats: We shield them from strangers, control the images and words they're exposed to on TV and computer screens, and keep antibacterial wipes within arm's reach in every room in the house. Yet, the biggest threat to our children may reside in our own kitchen cabinets.

The results speak for themselves:

- In the past thirty years, childhood obesity has tripled, and today, one in three kids is obese or overweight.
- Less than one-third of all children aged six to seventeen engage in vigorous activity.
- High blood pressure, type 2 diabetes, and high cholesterol—once thought to be diseases of the aging—are now diagnosed in elementary school children and teens.
- An estimated 33 percent of U.S. adults twenty years and older are overweight; 34 percent are obese, and 6 percent are extremely obese.

It's easy to blame society, the government, and the food industry for the problems our children face. And hey, it's easier and cheaper to eat crappy food—especially in tough economic times. But caring enough to wake our kids up, get them to school, clothe them, take them to soccer practice, and pay for piano lessons isn't enough. Kids learn by watching us. And in the long run, they'll eat what we eat, drink what we drink, and be as active as we are.[1]

Working out sucks . . . but raising unhealthy kids sucks more. It's a jungle out there, and leaving your kids ill equipped physically is as bad as, or worse than, letting them fall behind the pack intellectually or socially.

SEAT BELTS, CIGARETTES, AND CHILDHOOD OBESITY

The factor that puts children at greatest risk of being overweight is having obese parents.

—MICHELLE L. BRANDT, "Obese Parents Increase Kids' Risk of Being Overweight," *Stanford Report*, July 21, 2004

Do we need to throw parents of obese kids in jail?

Before you dismiss that question as unrealistic or outlandish, consider that child abuse and neglect are crimes that can get parents locked up and children placed in foster care. In fact, in a controversial 2011 opinion piece in the revered *Journal of the American Medical Association*, David Ludwig, a physician and researcher at the Harvard-affiliated Children's Hospital Boston, claimed that putting extremely obese children in foster care is arguably more ethical than obesity surgery: "[State intervention] ideally will support not just the child but the whole family, with the goal of re-uniting child and family as soon as possible. That may require instruction on parenting."

With the exception of rare medical conditions, obesity in kids is a definite symptom of abuse or neglect. Especially for kids who grow up in low-income families—where the cheapness and accessibility of junk food make it ubiquitous in the home—childhood obesity is a reversible condition that can be resolved with proper nutrition and exercise.[1]

So how do we get parents to change—how do we impose the most effective disincentive? Fine them? Raise their taxes? Give them a ticket if their kids tip the scale?

Consider the successful strategy of seat belts and cigarettes. For years, antismoking and seat belt campaigns were initiated using various educational and marketing scare tactics. But meaningful results did not occur until legal and financial consequences were set: Adults are now severely penalized if they are caught selling cigarettes to minors or not making their kids wear seat belts. Don't buckle up? Get a traffic ticket. Sell cigarettes to a minor? Get fined or lose your job. We see the residual benefit of both scenarios when kids turn to their parents and ask, "Why are you smoking?" and "Why aren't you buckling up?"

But when it comes to kids' health and nutrition, where are the meaningful consequences of failure? I have yet to see a parent get arrested or receive a ticket when his or her kid develops type 2 diabetes.

It's easy to blame school lunch ladies, vending machines, and video games for fattening our kids. But we need to put the responsibility where it truly belongs: on moms and dads.

Working out sucks . . . but leading an entire generation into a shorter life span and lower quality of life sucks even more. Obesity-related costs are currently the number one expense in the healthcare system, and baby boomer parenting has clearly babied us too much. If you want people to change, make it hurt if they don't—that's human nature. You have the right to remain sedentary, but I wouldn't recommend it.

iDEATH

The current generation is on track to have a shorter lifespan than their parents, and by 2048, all American adults will be overweight or obese.

—PRESIDENT'S COUNCIL ON FITNESS, SPORTS AND NUTRITION, AND THE CENTERS FOR DISEASE CONTROL AND PREVENTION

I admire Apple. I enjoy its ads. And I love its products. It's too bad the company is killing us.

Okay, the geniuses at Apple aren't exactly killing us, but they're sure making it easier for us to do it ourselves. Consider this: The leading cause of death in the United States—for both men and women and among all ethnic groups—is cardiovascular disease (CVD). It outranks cancer, stroke, chronic respiratory diseases, suicides, homicides, HIV/AIDS, and all unintentional or accidental deaths. CVD doesn't just kill the elderly; it's the leading cause of death for all Americans aged thirty-five and older, with over one million fatalities each year. A number of behaviors practiced by people every day contribute markedly to CVD, but lack of physical activity is chief among them. "So what?" you say. "Another person has a heart attack. We read about it every day. It won't happen to me."

Well, as we all know, technology is the great enabler. What is going to happen to an entire generation of people who succumb to serious screen addiction—not just their phones, but TV, video games, tablet computers, and whatever's coming next? If you consider all the threats to our country—terrorism, global warming, natural disasters, war, economic depressions—you can't help but wonder: Has technology (and the luxury it provides) become our own worst enemy? Is holding a smartphone to your head any different from holding a gun to your head? When should we start wearing pink ribbons for those who have been killed by Sitting Disease?[1]

The stats back it up: We're experiencing a slow societal decay brought on by rampant consumerism, hyper-immediate gratification, ubiquitous access to cheap junk food, and addictions to screens that promote sedentary lives. Coupled with poor nutrition, our choice to ignore physical activity has burrowed into our lives and become our own cancer—a self-inflicted genocide that has only begun to play out and will continue to spread over the following decades unless we change. Indeed, our own worst enemy lies within. (And inside the Apple Store.)

Working out sucks . . . but CVD sucks more. The cliché is true: You're either part of the problem or part of the solution. And if you lead, others will follow. You can choose to live like a zombie, addicted to glowing computer, TV, and iPad screens, or you can engage in a meaningful relationship with yourself, get healthy, and create the tipping point that sparks serious change. Hey, if nothing else, you'll have hotter photos of yourself to share on Facebook . . . using your iPhone app.

DOES GARFIELD HAVE
THE FAT GENE?

A quick aside: A recent report in *USA Today* states that two-thirds of our pets are now considered obese.

Did I miss something?

When did dogs start playing video games? When did we start lacing our cat food with high-fructose corn syrup? Have hamsters fallen prey to Internet porn addiction? Do fish need to eat more . . . um, fish? And when does the awareness campaign for Pet Obesity Month begin? Go figure; October 13 is the National Pet Obesity Awareness Day. (You can't make this stuff up!) [1]

> *Pet obesity is now the biggest health threat to pets in the US.*
> *The costs of obesity in illness and injury make it the number one*
> *medical issue seen in today's veterinary hospitals.*
> —ERNEST WARD JR., DVM, Association for Pet Obesity Prevention

You know the idea of a canary in a coal mine: If a canary dies in a mining tunnel, the miners know that the noxious gases will eventually kill them, too. Pet obesity is almost the reverse. Like the state of our kids, the state of our pets reflects our problematic lifestyles. We're already unhealthy and overweight. Now our cats and dogs (and maybe even our canaries) are proving the old adage that pets and pet owners eventually do start to look alike—unfortunately for the pets.

Working out sucks . . . but having an obese pet sucks more; it's animal cruelty. You feed them, bathe them, and provide vaccinations. They are 100 percent dependent, so when it comes to their health and welfare, there's no one else to blame. (Kind of like being a parent, but at least we can blame vending machines and school lunch ladies for fattening our kids, right?)

GOOD FOR YOUR IQ, BAD FOR YOUR GQ

Take something you love to do, mix it with something you hate to do, and what happens? The hate infects the love and destroys the pleasure.

That's why I've never understood why people try to read while exercising. I'll see them holding a paperback, struggling to turn the pages—all while walking at a very slow pace. Look, if you can read a book and exercise at the same time, you aren't exercising hard enough. Exercise should make you sweat, and if it doesn't cause labored breathing, you need to challenge yourself more.

Plus, reading during exercise can injure you. Over the years, I've seen plenty of treadmillers veer to the side, fall off the back, or lose their footing on their way to a face plant or an ass plant. It's not only embarrassing, but also painful. In fact about a year ago, an older woman tried to make an insurance claim against a fitness club after she suffered an injury while reading on the treadmill (probably the same woman who sued McDonald's over its hot coffee). Once the insurance company found out the facts, it challenged the member and never paid a cent.

Working out sucks . . . but letting it make everything else suck, sucks more. Hey, it's only thirty minutes. You can live without reading that book, writing that text, or flipping through Ashton Kutcher's tweets. And if you're the guy working out next to me wearing that ridiculous Bluetooth gear and carrying on self-important conversations loud enough for the entire club to hear, be prepared to have that earpiece bitch-slapped off your head. Unless you're the president of the United States, you're not that busy.

GEKKO AND GEICO

I'm an avid believer in personal responsibility, and I'm reluctant to suggest that the government needs to get involved
in the personal fitness and nutrition habits of individuals.
But I'm also a pragmatist, and let's face it: Personal responsibility went out of fashion with bell bottoms and the Bee
Gees. In the business arena, we structure compensation
plans to incentivize employee behavior, and it works. Gor-
don Gekko was partially right when he said, "Greed is good.
Greed works."

So the truth is this: If we want to alter the behavior of an
entire society, we need to provide a financial carrot. Yes, it's
unfortunate that people need monetary incentives to be
healthy, but money changes behavior faster than education—
and the simple solution of better physical health will not
only insulate against societal decay, but also advance us to a
better family, community, and planet tomorrow.

It's already working. In Minnesota, where Anytime Fitness is headquartered, the four largest health insurance
providers subsidize fitness memberships by reimbursing
insured customers twenty dollars per month if they use a
local health club at least twelve times a month. Our stats
have indicated a 55 percent usage rate, which is 20 percent
higher than normal usage and one of the best rates in the

fitness industry (normally, only one out of every three members uses a club that often).

Which brings me to GEICO. You've seen the commercials and heard the phrase "Fifteen minutes can save you 15 percent or more on car insurance." The ads are clever, and GEICO spends over $500 million a year drilling its message into our heads. But TV ad memorability is not the only secret to the company's success. It's also the fact that we have more control over our car insurance than we do over, say, health insurance. Most of us make conscious choices to drive within the speed limit, obey traffic laws, wear a seat belt, maintain a clean driving record, and make other lifestyle choices (own a home, get good grades, join AAA) to lower our auto-insurance costs.

We work hard to be good drivers, because, unlike health insurance, all of the money for car insurance comes directly out of our pockets.

When it comes to health insurance, we've never cared much about our choices, because employers paid the premium. Not anymore. With the unending rise in health-care expenses, employers are shifting more costs to their employees. In fact, companies are often reluctant to hire, because their employee benefits cost them almost fifty cents for every dollar of employee wages. The upside: Once people feel the pain in their own wallets, they adopt healthier lifestyles—just like auto insurance. I can't wait for the day when a commercial says: "Fifteen minutes can save you 15 percent or more on health insurance!"

Working out sucks . . . but paying more and more of your skyrock-
eting health insurance premiums sucks more. If you think you
won't be affected, you're wrong. Employers are implementing wellness plans, and if you don't engage, you'll pay more. It's your
choice: Lose the fat, or lose your money.

MONEY IS ALLERGIC
TO FAT PEOPLE

There is another consequence to packing on extra weight: being fat costs money—tens of thousands of dollars over a lifetime. Heavy people do not spend more than normal-size people on food, but their life insurance premiums are two to four times as large. They can expect higher medical expenses, and they tend to make less money and accumulate less wealth in their shortened lifetimes. They can have a harder time being hired, and then a harder time winning plum assignments and promotions.

—DAMON DARLIN, "Extra Weight, Higher Costs,"
New York Times, December 2, 2006

While we're on the topic of money, don't we all dream of winning the lottery? Of course we do. And none of us will. If you really want to get rich, the statistics say that you should start caring for your health. People who work out three to four times a week have a higher average annual income than those who don't work out regularly. Why? Because exercise takes discipline, hard work, goal-setting, and accountability. And these traits are monetized in the business arena.[1]

I've found that attorneys, doctors, and engineers are the people who complete marathons and triathlons, because their professions require independent hard work. For these people, pushing themselves is second nature. They're willing to make the sacrifice to succeed in both work and play.

Workers who are in better shape also make more money and get promoted more often than their obese coworkers. Consider that each of us is a brand. As an employer, do you want to promote a brand that's out of shape (which might convey laziness and lack of discipline) or a brand that represents energy, hard work, time management, self-control, and better health?

Being fat is also expensive—for individuals, especially women, and all of society. In a study at George Washington University, researchers added in things like employee sick days, lost productivity, and even the need for extra gasoline and found that the annual cost of being obese is $4,879 for a woman and $2,646 for a man.

Plus, inactivity and obesity-related illnesses are choking our health-care system and leading us down a path where the healthy pay for the unhealthy. That's tolerable as long as "the unhealthy" are a minority. But what's going to happen in 2020, when over 80 percent of adults are projected to be obese? The redistribution of wealth may not be able to tolerate the redistribution of girth.

Working out sucks . . . but making less money than your healthier peers sucks a lot more. Think about your bottom the next time you're looking at your bottom line. And if you want to be wealthy, start getting healthy. You won't be discriminated against, you'll see an immediate savings in daily living expenses, and you'll have more opportunities than ever before.

GENETICS SUCK

A friend of mine attended a community exercise gathering in the park. It was a free event that invited families to learn more about eating better, preparing healthy meals, and encouraging physical activities for the entire family. She brought her five-year-old daughter, and at one point, the little girl asked her out of the blue, "Mommy, does God like fat people?" Embarrassed, the mother quickly responded in a quiet voice, "Of course honey. God loves everyone." To which the daughter replied, "Then why did he make them so big?"

Some people think there's such a thing as a fat gene; others don't. I say, *who cares?*

Yes, there are some things we can't control when it comes to how we look, think, and behave. I've seen it over twenty years in the fitness industry: Some people have to work four times harder to get the half the results. Some folks can eat endless amounts of junk food and carbs without adding a pound to their delicate bone structure while others can put on cellulite just by looking at a menu. I empathize with people who are always running into a fitness headwind, but you have to accept that you didn't win the genetic lottery, and work with what you've been given.

Am I about to use that tired phrase uttered by so many motivational gurus: "You can do anything you set your mind to"? No, that's crap. No matter how hard I could have worked, my NBA playing days ended when my dad's sperm united with my mom's egg. Done. *Finito*. Airball. And no matter how hard some people work, they'll never become a rock star, the president of the United States, or Angelina Jolie. When it comes to personal fitness, most of us will never look like an "after" photo.

But here's the thing: The after photo isn't the end game. The goal is to have more energy, feel better about yourself, and live a fuller, more complete life—period. If you can do that, it's a slam dunk.

Working out sucks . . . but self-pity sucks more. If you have to work harder than others to achieve results, embrace it. They need to run a mile; you need to run three. They can eat pizza every week; you can treat yourself once a month. So be it. Quit comparing yourself with fitness models and buff celebrities in *People* magazine, and face the facts: Self-pity doesn't burn calories.

2:03:02

During the 2011 Boston Marathon, Geoffrey Mutai posted an astonishing time of 2:03:02. That equates to an average speed of nearly *thirteen miles per hour for just over two hours—each mile under five minutes.* It's difficult to comprehend running at that speed for over twenty-six miles, but it just goes to show you what the body and mind can achieve.

In 1897, the first-ever Boston Marathon was completed in 2:55:10. Over the course of 114 years, human beings have managed to shave off fifty-two minutes, eight seconds. That's the same race in 30 percent less time. Running a sub-four-minute mile was once thought to be impossible. Now it's so common that it doesn't even make the news.

What has changed? Have our hearts and lungs grown in capacity by 30 percent? Are we born with 30 percent more muscle? Has the human body experienced any significant physiological changes in the last hundred years, or have we simply learned to train better, eat smarter, and recover more quickly?

To me, the answer is simple: Competition, personal motivation, and a deeper understanding about our bodies have pushed us past the boundaries of our own expectations.

I've already written about being more realistic. But here's the flip side of that argument: If you think you're already pushing yourself to your physical limits, think again. With proper, consistent training, your body can handle almost anything you throw at it. But what about your mind?

The real challenge is overcoming your own excuses—the process that used to be called willpower. You might not care about running a marathon (I don't), but everyone has an inner motivation that can be enhanced with increased levels of fitness. What's your *personal* motivation to put down that bag of chips, to get off the couch, and to get moving? To be more attractive? To be able to play with your kids? To save money on your health insurance?

I know the motivation is there, because you're reading this book. The question is, are you listening to it?

Working out sucks . . . but refusing to challenge yourself sucks more. You may never run the Boston Marathon, but think of the finish line as your desired lifestyle destination. It's there for the taking. Your body and mind can get you there. Just take the first step.

FRIENDS CAN SUCK, TOO

Achieving success in almost any endeavor is more difficult to do as a solo act, and I don't just say that because of Steve Perry's post-Journey career.

Consider the strategy used in behavioral therapy for addicts, where the treatment includes regular group meetings and an assigned mentor to help you through your recovery process. This safety net provides support and motivation, and helps you fight the temptations that lurk around every corner and in the shadows of your mind.

This strategy also works as you pursue your fitness goals. If you can find a friend, family member, or coworker with similar goals and a high level of motivation, you'll be pushed to exercise harder and get your butt to the club when you don't want to go. It's easy to blow off working out if it's just you; but if Dick and Jane are waiting for you to show up, you're more likely to stick to it. And as your buddy's partner, you can do your part by holding him or her accountable, too. I've seen this work thousands of times for mothers and daughters, fathers and sons, coworkers, cousins, husbands and wives, best friends, and people who just met in the weight room.

But here's the thing: Be careful who you choose as a workout partner, because it can easily go the wrong way.

Sometimes, friends, family members, and coworkers will unintentionally (or intentionally) sabotage your personal wellness pursuits out of insecurity and fear that you'll get in good shape and leave them behind. You see, if lazy, out-of-shape people surround themselves with lazy, out-of-shape people, they don't feel so lazy and out of shape. But every time you work out, they're reminded how lazy and out of shape they are. So some people will try to keep you down. They'll talk you out of working out, and before you know it, you're in a movie theater holding a bathtub of buttered pop-corn and a keg of soda that would satiate a rhino. If you're showing any weakness (which all of us do), it's easy to blow off the workout and promise you'll start eating healthier: "Monday after the weekend, and this time, I'm serious!" But you won't, and you know it.

Working out sucks . . . but shared laziness sucks more. You can't change a bad habit into a good one without the right safety net and support network. Find a health partner who has similar goals, schedules, and lifestyles—and make it fun by creating contests, ex-ercising outside, trying new training routines, splitting the cost of a trainer, or sharing iPod playlists. You can "just do it" all you want; but don't do it alone (or with a friend who's really just an enabler).

SUPERMAN HAD KRYPTONITE; OPRAH HAD MAC 'N' CHEESE

Everybody knows that TV fuels a sedentary lifestyle. But there's an even more sinister way in which we let the flat screen make us rounder. I'm going to start by targeting Oprah Winfrey, so first, a disclaimer:

Oprah, I admire the hell out of you. You've been one of the most influential people of the last twenty years. You've brought dignity and class to daytime TV. You've sparked newfound interest in how our bodies work (Dr. Oz), as well as in interior design, style, food, and countless other subjects. And you've single-handedly raised the level of literacy and book sales with your book club. There. Now I can get to the "but." Because, Oprah, in one important way, you let us—and yourself—down.

Oprah has always been refreshingly frank about her weight, and an out-of-synch thyroid condition has exacerbated the problem. But remember 1988? She stepped on stage in her size 10 Calvin Klein jeans and black turtleneck, and millions of us took in the indelible image of Skinny Oprah. It was one of her all-time highest-rated shows. She had lost over 60 pounds from dieting, and millions of viewers were instantly inspired to eat better and exercise more—even though she later admitted that her strict low-calorie diet was unsustainable.

In the years since, Oprah's yo-yo dieting has caused her weight to fluctuate to between 167 and 237 pounds, and while we've identified with her battle, we've also lost hope in ourselves. The perception has become this: If Oprah Winfrey—with the money to hire the best nutritionists, chefs, personal trainers, and doctors in the world—can't do it, then how can I? Americans have a tendency to think that money can buy anything, so if we see somebody rich failing to achieve a goal . . . well, that's it. Stick a fork in us—and then stick a fork in the buttered mashed potatoes.

That's one side of the TV screen. Then there's what appears to be the opposite: the increasing number of shows that feature real people, "just like us," who actually do win the weight battle (think *The Biggest Loser* and other health-related reality shows). These are positive influences, right?

Wrong. Here we have an entirely different trap: In the course of a single sixty-minute episode, we watch contestants lose 50, 100, 200, or even 300 or more pounds. The effect misleads us into thinking that we should be losing significantly more weight each week than what our scale tells us, and in a world ruled by immediate gratification, we lose hope and motivation when we don't experience immediate de-fatification. This frustration leads to stress, shame, and disappointment, which undermines our motivation and triggers emotional eating. Because we don't have the benefit of living in a time-lapse world with the best editors Hollywood can buy, we give up the hope of ever losing weight on our own without being monitored 24/7 by trainers, nutritionists, and doctors. In this situation, we are fooled by "un-reality TV." And as you may have gathered from the chapters you've read so far, this book isn't here to reinforce the bull-shit. It's here to remind you that . . .

Working out sucks . . . but if your weight-loss strategy is dictated by a celebrity (or you're waiting to be chosen for a reality TV show), that sucks even more. Money can't buy a healthy body, and the fight to eat healthier and exercise regularly is a constant struggle for most people—even the supersmart, super wealthy celebrity who has access to the best support groups in the world. It's going to be a difficult, personal challenge, but you're not a failure if you don't achieve it; you're a failure only if you don't try. So turn off the TV and get started—or get on an elliptical machine and burn some calories *while* you watch Oprah!

THE $600 COAT HANGER

Remember when financial experts were predicting that traditional brick-and-mortar retailing was going to shrivel up and die? That the Internet was going to let everyone stay home and buy everything online? Today, people can order almost anything (even groceries) while sitting on a couch in a Snuggie and, in many cases, buy it at a lower price and with free shipping. Yet traditional retailing is as strong as ever. What happened? The financial experts underestimated the experience of touching the sweaters, smelling the mangos, strapping on the high heels, and hearing the holiday music.

It's a little like going to a bar versus staying at home. At home, the drinks are considerably cheaper, and you don't have to wait in line to pee. Yet we still go to bars. Why? Because of the atmosphere and social connection.

It's no different with exercise equipment. Infomercials always make it sound so tempting to buy a huge hunk of metal (or one of those gimmicky padded springy things always promoted by Suzanne Somers) to get you looking like Brad Pitt or Jennifer Aniston in thirty days. Going to the neighborhood gym three or four times a week? That's for suckers! You can hit the treadmill before work or burn off an entire day's calories while watching *Seinfeld* reruns after the kids go to bed. It makes logical sense and appears easy—and nothing could be more convenient than working out in your home, right?

Wrong. You don't have a chance. You've failed before you started. And you're wasting your money. Why? Let me count the ways.

Because the couch is a fiercer competitor than the treadmill.

Because you should really call your mom back.

Because the lawn needs fertilizing.

Because your kids need extra help with their homework.

Because bedtime is taking longer than usual.

Because your spouse wants to cuddle and eat ice cream.

Because you need to answer 150 unopened e-mails.

Because it sounds a lot more fun to share vacation photos on Facebook.

Because you just need to rest and put your feet up for a few minutes.

Because using the same piece of equipment over and over again will slow results and bore you into quitting.

Because the atmosphere of your home is about comfort and relaxation, not high-energy exercise.

Need I go on? Listen, home is great for most things, but it sucks for exertion. Every time you think about working out, the devil on your shoulder is going to whisper "TV," "couch," "computer," "fridge," "kids," "quiet time," "reading," "scrapbooking" or "*SportsCenter*." Don't fall into the trap.

Working out sucks . . . but setting yourself up for failure sucks more. Don't play against impossible odds, and don't waste your money on a $600 treadmill that will eventually serve as a coat hanger before it appears on eBay or Craigslist for half its original value.

I LOVE MILFS!

Get your mind out of the gutter. I mean that I love Mothers Into Lifelong Fitness.

Statistically speaking, women aren't as physically strong as men. But you and I know the truth: When it comes to determination, pain tolerance, and discipline, estrogen beats the crap out of testosterone every time. Take moms. When it comes to their children, mothers of many species will literally give their lives to raise or protect their offspring. In my career, I've seen a lot more female success stories than male. And if a married couple succeeds in dramatically changing their health together, chances are the effort was led by the wife.

Statistics prove that healthy parents typically raise healthy children. If even just one parent is obese, a child has a 60 percent chance of being obese. If both parents are overweight, that chance increases to 80 percent.
—STANFORD UNIVERSITY MEDICAL REPORT ON OBESITY

But I've also seen mothers use children as an excuse not to get in shape. A lot of moms feel guilty about working out, seeing it as a selfish pursuit of their personal fitness at the expense of their kids. But here's the thing: To be a great mom, you need to be a healthy mom. You need energy. You need to feel good about yourself. You need to keep up with your kids and be a role model. You need to disconnect from work, chores, helping with homework, and being a soccer chauffeur—and simply plug into "me time."[1]

> *Mothers are commonly viewed as role models for eating behavior and serve as the gatekeepers of food. Empowering and educating women is the best way we know to break the cycle of obesity and promote healthy habits for the life of any woman and her loved ones.*
>
> —ELIZABETH BATTAGLINO CAHILL, RN, executive director of HealthyWomen

A lot of moms tell me that they feel tired, overwhelmed, and too busy—and they lack the willpower or discipline to work out. I remind them that as a mom, they've most likely already survived some or all of the following:

- Nine-plus months of turbulent physical and emotional changes during pregnancy;
- A long stretch of time during which they had to stop drinking alcohol, limit caffeine intake, monitor their diet, and stay away from secondhand smoke;
- Morning sickness, swollen legs, poor circulation, fluctuating hormones, overall discomfort, and internal pressure on their bladder making them pee every ten minutes;
- The aftereffects of pregnancy, including weight gain, stretch marks, and varicose veins;
- The immense pain of birth itself, which no man can even begin to imagine.

So my question is, if you've already successfully altered your life for a child, why can't you do it for yourself?

Working out sucks . . . but moms don't. In fact, they rule. If you're a mom who can't summon the inspiration to be a MILF, then either you're underestimating yourself, or you've forgotten just how strong you can be. Tap into that steely resolve, and do it for yourself or your children or so you can make all your friends (and ex-boyfriends) envious. That last motivation can be particularly gratifying . . .

DUDE,
GET YOUR HARD ON!

In the interest of equal time, let me talk bluntly to the men for a second.

Listen, Dude, dozens of studies have documented how often you think about sex. Some say it's multiple times a week; others say it's every seven seconds. Whatever it is, let's simply agree on one thing: You think about sex all the freakin' time. Well, guess what? More exercise equals more sex. Can you hear me now?

Here are some other things proven by studies. People who exercise not only have sex more often, but also perform better. Exercise helps sexual aging, reduces erectile dysfunction, and makes people feel more sexually attractive. Still listening?

All of this makes sense, because sex and exercise are physiological cousins. During both activities, your body releases endorphins. Have you heard the term *runner's high?* The feeling of bliss and contentment that a seasoned runner may experience during exercise is caused by a massive endorphin orgy. Your sex drive and feelings of sexual pleasure also use an endorphin release system. Each time you exercise, your body releases these endorphins. The more frequent and intense the releases, the easier it is for sexual

arousal and pleasure in the future. In fact, women who frequently exercise become aroused more quickly and are able
to reach orgasm faster and more intensely. (More motivation to get your significant other to exercise with you, because . . . well, do you really think you're having too much
sex, already?)

Plus, if you're physically fit, you may have more options
for sex. Sex may sometimes be an intense physical activity
requiring strength and endurance. As you exercise, your
strength and stamina will increase, opening the possibility
for more varied sexual positions that require greater physical control. (Scan those last two paragraphs again: Women
. . . arousal . . . orgasm . . . strength . . . stamina . . . sexual
positions.)

Okay, moving on from sex. The truth is, men need regular
physical activity for a variety of reasons. High cholesterol
puts men at increased risk for heart attacks, strokes, and pe-
ripheral artery disease. For many of us, the risk of high cholesterol starts in our twenties and increases with age.
Genetics plays a role, but a variety of lifestyle factors, including diet, activity level, and body weight, also affect cholesterol levels. Plus, men are reporting higher stress levels
due to high and sometimes competing expectations from
both work and home. In general, men tend to bottle up their
feelings (big surprise). And in turn, stress causes irregular
sleeping patterns, irritability, high blood pressure, weight
gain, relationship changes, fatigue, depression, and low sex
drive. What's the best prescription to alleviate stress? Regular exercise, a smart nutrition plan, and regular sleep—after
sex, of course.

Working out sucks . . . but not having sex sucks more. When it comes to gaining confidence, alleviating stress, lowering cholesterol, and actually doing that certain thing that you think about every seven seconds—and doing it well—exercise is a mental and physical Viagra.

FOOD DOES NOT SUCK

I'm a carnivore. I love a big, juicy steak. And downing a hamburger loaded with onions, jalapeños, cheese, and a fried egg served with a side of french fries and a chocolate malt is a sexual experience without the wet spot. The thought of ice cream turns me into Pookie from the movie *New Jack City*. In fact, if ice cream were a wife, I'd be a polygamist in the church of Baskin-Robbins. Should I go on?

My point is this: I understand the love affair with tantalizing food, so I won't try to convince you to eat tofu burgers and rice cakes. But nutrition is just as important as—if not more important than—exercise when it comes to weight control, energy levels, and mood swings.

The problem is, there's a war going on when it comes to food. We're mostly at war with ourselves and our temptations, but our health is also at war with the diabolical marketers of the Evil Food Empire. Their weapons include slick ads, huge or deceptive serving sizes, and high-calorie ingredients hidden like so many Greek soldiers inside a flabby Trojan horse.[1]

These neverending seductions, coupled with the alarming statistics on obesity and diabetes (already mentioned in this book), are enough to make you wonder: When it comes to national security, does our biggest threat reside in a desert in Afghanistan or on every street corner in America (not to mention in our own refrigerators)? Who kills more people: terrorists or the Junk Food Jihad? We already tore down the statue of Saddam Hussein; should Ronald McDonald be next?

Consider these alarming facts compiled from the *Fooducate* and *Healthy Meal Experts* Web sites:

- In 1970, Americans spent $6 billion a year on fast food. Today, it's over $110 billion.
- That's more money than we spend on higher education, personal computers, computer software, or new cars.
- That's also more money than we spend on movies, books, magazines, newspapers, videos, and recorded music combined.
- The average weight for a female in the early 1960s was 140.2 pounds. In the 1990s, that figure increased to 164.3 pounds. For men, it swelled from 166 to 191.3.
- Twenty years ago, a typical hamburger packed 333 calories. Today, 590. Pizza has gone from 500 calories a slice to 850.

Worse yet is when an item is marketed as healthy when it's really laden with frivolous calories (not to mention mounds of sugar and salt). Take McDonald's oatmeal. Sounds healthy, right? But factor in the cream or brown sugar, and you might as well order the cheesy breakfast burrito.

This kind of sneaky stuff happens in all types of "healthy" marketed food. When you grab a bag of 100-calorie snacks or a low-fat dessert, have you ever looked to see how many servings make up 100 calories and how many total servings are in a bag? That's where the food marketers get you, because if 3.5 chips make up 100 calories, who the hell stops after eating 3.5 chips? So after feed-bagging yourself a pouch of low-fat rice cakes, don't be too proud: You've still probably consumed 500 calories, which may equate to a quarter of your recommended daily intake.

Yes, we are stuffing our faces with high-caloric junk food and getting fat. And yes, it's easy to blame food companies. But we still live in a free country. We still have choices. And there are plenty of options for smart, healthy, low-calorie meals that offer nutritional balance and still taste good. Plus, whatever happened to moderation? When did dessert become an everyday thing? Why are kids being given treats after every gathering—T-ball games, birthday parties, movie time, or for just doing ordinary kid stuff? Our parenting techniques are starting to mirror the dolphin trainers at Sea World: Every time our son or daughter does a freakin' somersault, we reward the kid with a bucket of sugary gum.

To understand how fitness and nutrition work, you only need to understand basic math. If you consume 2,000 calories a day, that equates to 14,000 a calories a week. A pound of fat is the equivalent of 3,500 calories, so to burn off one pound a week, you need to burn off 17,500 calories in that week (14,000 + 3,500). If you consume more than you burn, you gain weight. It's that simple. Now consider that a cupcake may have 500 calories. For most people, that's the equivalent of jogging on a treadmill for forty minutes. Is that five-minute enjoyment from a cupcake really worth forty minutes of sweat?

Working out sucks . . . but losing the food war sucks more. Let's get back to common sense. Treat yourself in moderation, and continue to enjoy even the high-calorie stuff—just not as much and not as often. Challenge yourself to cook meals with vegetables, unprocessed food, fruit, and lean cuts of meat. Teach yourself and your kids to pay attention to what they're putting in their mouths and stomachs. And stop being so damn gullible (or willfully ignorant) about claims of low-fat or healthy food. If a food makes a health claim, the food probably isn't healthy. So if you really believe that a bowl of Froot Loops gives you your recommended daily number of fruit servings, then you probably deserve the nickname "Cankles."

COOKING THE BOOKS

In the previous chapter, I talked about how sneaky food marketers disguise caloric intake with slick labels and cleverly determined portion sizes. Here's another secret: Most restaurants significantly underreport the calories in their meals.

Don't freak. I'm not going to discourage you from eating out, because that's simply not realistic. Restaurants provide an intoxicating combination of great food, atmosphere, and relationship nurturing—and frankly, eating out has replaced baseball as our national pastime.

> *According to* Restaurants USA *magazine,*
> *Americans eat out for 4.2 meals per week.*

But you need to know that your meals are likely bloated with more calories than you think. The USDA Human Nutrition Research Center on Aging at Tufts University recently sent a team of scientists to purchase items from over forty-two fast-food and sit-down eateries in Indiana, Arkansas, and Massachusetts—including Burger King, Olive Garden, Outback Steakhouse, McDonald's, Taco Bell, and Chuck E. Cheese.[1] Then they measured the actual calories these items contained. Here's what they discovered:

- Only 7 percent of the 269 foods tested were within 10 calories of their reported numbers.
- Almost 20 percent packed at least 100 calories more than what was indicated.
- The biggest discrepancies occurred in sit-down restaurants, where the stated calorie count for a menu item was off by an average of 225 calories.
- At fast-food restaurants, the average discrepancy was 134 calories per menu item.

Remember, weight loss is simple math: If you consume more than you burn, you gain weight. As the study's lead author, Susan Roberts, noted, "Over the course of a year, an extra 100 calories daily can add up to 10 to 15 pounds." In other words, if you think the low-fat lasagna is a smart choice because it's listed on the "under 500 calories" menu, think again. An extra 250 calories cancels out your thirty-minute morning exercise routine, and over the course of a year . . . well, let's just say, there's more than one reason it's called eating "out."

Working out sucks . . . but letting restaurants become a menu for disaster sucks more. You don't need to stop running for the border or cancel your son's Chuck E. Cheese birthday-palooza. Just make a commitment to educating yourself about food when you're at a restaurant, and don't be afraid to grill the waiter about the grilled chicken.

SOUL CALORIES

Contrary to what you might think, my motivation for writing this book isn't to create some utopian society filled with people who look like Ken and Barbie. But you must accept that physical appearance is a global currency that shows no signs of weakening. Plastic surgery (for both men and women) is a growing, multibillion-dollar industry—and we spend billions more on makeup, shoes, clothing, and accessories. The fitness industry is obsessed with promising bodily nirvana in the form of glorious glutes, rambunctious rhomboids, delicious deltoids, and other fetishized muscle groups. Every infomercial is inundated with the before-and-after pictures of the chubby hubby who magically transformed into "The Rock."

Everyone wants to look better on the outside, but what happens on the inside when you exercise regularly? Let me try to describe the feeling. Think back to some of the bigger projects you've completed in your life: repainting a room in your home, creating a garden, completing a lengthy report for high school or college, or finishing an important project at work. Or even consider smaller tasks, like mowing your lawn, organizing your garage, or helping your son or daughter finish a school science project. Each of these tasks took serious effort, but you were gratified by a sense of accomplishment and pride when it was over. When you finish something—even something as routine as mowing the lawn—seeing the completed task makes you feel better about yourself.

This is the same feeling you get after every single work-out. It's like taking a syringe of energy and self-confidence and injecting it into your body three or four times per week. And while vanity may provide the initial motivation, it's the internal reward—the regular dose of accomplishment and pride—that turns regular people into fitness addicts.

Another important benefit to regular exercise is stress relief, and over the years, countless fitness enthusiasts have described their workouts as "therapy" or "cleansing experiences." Let's agree that life isn't getting any less stressful. We have demanding jobs and increasing expectations as parents, students, or spouses. Plus, we're surrounded by uncontrollable external factors like economic recessions, natural disasters, mounting debt (on all fronts), and the omnipresent virtual connectedness of today's way of living. If stress were a stock, I'd load my portfolio with this appreciating asset.

To see further evidence that exercise provides a therapeutic and cleansing experience and alleviates stress, consider these surprising facts:

- In February 2011, a 6.3 earthquake rocked the city of Christchurch, New Zealand. Three months later, many of the businesses were still closed. The Anytime Fitness club suffered minor damage and was closed for one day. But since the quake, the club has experienced a significant increase in membership, reaching 1,350 members (350 people joined in one month).

- Hurricane Katrina was the costliest natural disaster in U.S. history. At Anytime Fitness, we offered additional support to our franchisees and made internal plans to anticipate club closures, long delays in reopening, and no new franchises to be sold or opened in southern Louisiana for a significant period. But guess what? The opposite happened. The majority of Louisiana clubs saw a surge of new enrollments, and franchise openings continued at a brisk pace. In fact, Louisiana was the second-fastest state to add Anytime Fitness clubs (after Minnesota) and still is to this day.
- After 9/11, the health clubs in and around New York City also reported a considerable spike in new membership enrollments.
- Through the last two major recessions with high periods of unemployment, health club memberships have either increased or shown no significant decline.

Please don't misinterpret this: I'm not celebrating the financial gain from tragic events. I'm simply drawing attention to the importance of stress relief and the therapeutic effect that regular exercise can provide. We shouldn't have to experience world calamities to avoid health catastrophes.

Working out sucks . . . but cellulite on the inside is far more damaging than the stuff on your thighs. Although the fitness industry is obsessed with perfect bodies, looking better is just a positive side effect of something much deeper. With every completed workout, you reduce stress and gain a sense of confidence, pride, energy, and accomplishment. And you provide healthy calories to feed your soul.

DO-IT-YOURSELF
ROOT CANAL?

For many people, health clubs fall into the category of things we love to hate. In fact, we share space with airlines, dentists, meteorologists, IRS agents, and octogenarians who still drive. Our industry doesn't help its cause, because over the last thirty years, we've fostered a reputation for high-pressure sales, stinky group–locker rooms, meathead trainers, and Britney Spears wannabe aerobics instructors wearing leg warmers and spandex. So why are all these insufferable things still in our lives?

Most people dislike the thought of flying, because after you get patted down like a teenager in the backseat at a drive-in, you have to shoehorn yourself next to a grumpy, overly talkative or super-plus-sized stranger. But if you're traveling a long distance, almost everyone still chooses to fly, because it saves valuable time.

Most people hate going to the dentist, because dentists are tooth-drilling sadists. (Heck, even dentists don't like going to the dentist.) But we understand the importance of our teeth for eating, smiling, and hygiene—and good dental care has actually been linked to longer life spans. So we begrudgingly visit the dentist, because he or she has the proper tools and training to care for our choppers. And hey, what's the alternative? Doing your own root canal?

A health club is no different. It's like driving versus flying, or like having nice teeth versus looking British. You can exercise on your own, but for a little more money, the fitness specialist will get you to your fitness destination much faster. Like the dentist, the health club is filled with specific tools—designed by knowledgeable engineers—to care for your body in a quick, safe, and effective manner. Furthermore, as mentioned in the introduction, there's a commercial fitness option for every type of person, pursuit, or budget. There are even niche clubs built for seniors, which might be where the octogenarian driver is driving to.

Working out sucks . . . but make it suck less by seeing a trained professional or choosing a fitness option that suits your lifestyle. A local fitness club will provide the education and variety needed to help you achieve progress, and if you experience faster results, you won't struggle with motivation.

(IT'S UP TO) YOU

Did you think I was exaggerating in some of the earlier chapters? Do you feel as if I'm blowing this fat issue out of proportion? Think again, because as I was writing these chapters, two similar articles were published within days of each other. The facts listed below not only support the message in this book, but also paint a depressing picture for generations to come. The bottom line: We'd better get *Working Out Sucks* translated into multiple languages, because this is not just a problem in the good ol' United States of McDonald's.

Nearly 10 percent of the world's adults have diabetes, and the prevalence of the disease is rising rapidly. As in the United States and other wealthy nations, increased obesity and inactivity are the primary cause in developing countries such as India, Latin America, the Caribbean and the Middle East. That's the sobering conclusion of a study published Saturday in the journal *Lancet* that traces trends in diabetes and average blood sugar readings in about 200 countries and regions over the past three decades. Its findings predict a huge burden of medical costs and physical disability lying ahead in this century, as diabetes increases a person's risk of heart attack, kidney failure, blindness and some infections.

"This study confirms the suspicion of many that diabetes has become a global epidemic," said Frank Hu, an epidemiologist at Harvard's School of Public Health who was not involved in the research. "It has the potential to overwhelm the health systems of many countries."

. . . Type 2 accounts for 90 percent of cases and generally comes on after age 25. It is controlled by insulin, pills and, in some cases, weight loss and exercise.

. . . "Diabetes tracks very well with economic development and urbanization," said Hu.[1]

(Sounds a lot like iDeath, doesn't it?) And another newspaper documents the state of fatness in all the states:

We're getting fatter. In 1995, no state had an obesity rate above 20 percent. Now, all but one does. An annual obesity report by two public health groups looked for the first time at state-by-state statistics over the last two decades.[2]

And another:

The number of people living with diabetes has soared to 366 million, and the disease kills one person every seven seconds, posing a "massive challenge" to healthcare systems worldwide. ... The vast majority of those with the disease have Type 2—the kind linked to poor diet, obesity and lack of exercise—and the problem is spreading as people in the developing world adopt more Western lifestyles. Diabetics have inadequate blood sugar control, which can lead to serious complications like heart disease and stroke, damage to the kidneys or nerves, and to blindness. Worldwide deaths from the disease are now running at 4.6 million a year. The latest figures, unveiled at the European Association for the Study of Diabetes (EASD) congress in Lisbon, underline the need for urgent action by governments ... according to top doctors in the field.[3]

Obese people now outnumber the undernourished and "excess nutrition now kills more than hunger."
—WORLD DISASTERS REPORT,
INTERNATIONAL FEDERATION OF THE RED CROSS

While these stats support the point of this book, I know you won't be motivated by global obesity rates or quotes from Harvard epidemiologists (I have no idea what that is, and I'm not going to Google it just to sound smart). But hopefully, you have found a personal reason—or multiple reasons—in this book to motivate yourself. Or at the very least, to stop accepting the lame, tired excuses of time or money.

I hope you take action to be a role model for your kids, to get a promotion at work, to have more sex, to not have the fattest dog in the park, to alleviate stress, to gain energy, to make jaws drop at your high school reunion, or to do your part for the greater good of an unfit society. Or, just do it for *you*. To experience a life with greater capacity, without the limitations of being overweight—and to live a life with more confidence, more smiles, and more fun.

Your life starts and ends with *you*, and one of the most powerful things you own is your ability to choose. Although you can't change yesterday, you do get to determine what to-morrow holds. And if you make the choice to be healthier, your newfound energy, motivation, and personal leadership will inspire friends, family, and coworkers. And the tipping point begins.

Working out sucks . . . but you don't, and your health is simply not negotiable. If you decide not to take action after reading this book, the good news is, you'll never feel guilt over your poor health again. You'll resign yourself to being out of shape, being constantly at risk for diabetes and heart disease, and being the person we dread seeing trudging toward us down the airplane aisle. You will have decided that your taste buds are more powerful than your brain and heart, and that your cravings for a Big Mac, a Snickers bar, or nine cans of Coke a day override your desires to live a life without labored breathing. You will have chosen to play with your kids less often, and you'll have decided to have less energy, have less sex, and make less money than your peers. Is that the case? Then put down this book, and head immediately to Walmart to buy elastic-waistband blue jeans and a fanny pack to fill with candy bars—and start saving money for one of those motorized shopping scooters.

Hopefully, you won't look back on your life with disappointment, because regret is the heaviest weight of all.

PART 2

CHANGING BEHAVIOR SUCKS, TOO, BUT . . .

We all know that working out sucks. And we sure know that nutrition sucks. Who wants to choose carrots over french fries, anyway? (You'll find more about nutrition in the next part of the book.)

The same is true for changing our behavior. Can an old dog (or an obese human) really learn new tricks?

Let's face it; we all have our very own secret (and not-so-secret) list of bad habits that we'd like to replace with healthier ones. But despite our best intentions, sometimes we don't succeed at breaking the perpetual cycle. We try every possible solution, offered or manufactured—only to end up with "(I Can't Get No) Satisfaction" playing on repeat in our minds.

When we fail to break a bad habit—whether it's eating a tub of ice cream in one sitting, smoking two packs a day, or fueling our minds with negative thoughts—we start to feel like a failure. It's as if we're climbing Mount Everest without hope of reaching the summit. We keep slipping on the rocks with bruised and battered bodies and egos, struggling to navigate through what feels like an impossible terrain.

But despite these uphill climbs and setbacks, there is a resiliency and an internal fortitude within all of us. In my twenty years of working with people, I've observed that we aren't stuck because we don't want to change; it's because we don't know how to change.

So, the answer is, "Yes, you can change your behavior . . . if you know how." In essence, we are all looking for a road map, a how-to guide to get us to the top of the mountain. I'm here to tell you there is hope—a magic bullet, so to say. Don't misunderstand me here, finding the bullet doesn't mean you won't have to work hard—really hard. But, with a few tools and solid direction, you can feel less stuck and start making life changes that will feel magical.

MIND OVER MATTER: A MAGICAL STORY OF CHANGE

In the fall of 2009, I met Tyler, a handsome and charming nineteen-year-old who was referred to me by his school counselor. This young man was the picture of success, at least on the outside: straight-A student, star athlete, social butterfly, and embarking on his freshman year in college, full ride scholarship in hand. As he shuffled in to my office, I couldn't help but notice his slumped shoulders, sad eyes, and glaring lack of confidence.

So, I started slowly: "How can I help you?"

After a long silence, he looked up and mumbled, "Something is wrong inside my head. I just see all the bad stuff—it's like there's an eraser that takes away everything good. I've tried to stop the eraser, but I can't."

He reached into his pocket and handed me a crumpled piece of paper.

"Here, take a look."

Drawn in black ink was a stick figure carrying an enormous backpack. The stick figure was hunched over, barely able to stand under the weight of the pack. The pack was bright red with the word PAIN written across the shoulder strap.

CHANGING BEHAVIOR SUCKS, TOO, BUT . . .

He looked me straight in the eye: "I was hoping you could help me burn my backpack."

When Tyler started his journey up the mountain, he saw himself as frail and powerless, carrying a backpack full of fear and negative thinking. He believed he was stupid, inadequate, and ugly. So ugly, he didn't want to live anymore. It didn't matter that other people told him he was capable and smart, he believed otherwise. Fear lurked everywhere— disappointing others, failing at school, looking stupid, getting laughed at, and being alone. Fear and pessimism had gotten the best of him, overshadowing his achievements and belief in the future. To relieve his pain, he had isolated himself in his dorm room, stopped doing his homework, and buried himself in the land of television and alcohol.

Eventually, Tyler grew tired of carrying his heavy pack and started looking for a solution. He found the courage to start facing his fears, one at a time.

"It's weird," he said. "This monster chases me everywhere. I can't seem to get away from it—like it's smarter than me."

"Tyler, what if you're smarter than the monster?"

"How's that gonna happen?"

I explained. "You'll have to separate your mind from your backpack."

"OK. What do you mean?"

For a fraction of a second, all I could see was confusion. "Hang on. This is how it works. Think of your backpack as your brain—the ultimate storage device. A huge sponge that soaks up everything you see, hear, touch, taste, and experience. Anything and everything you've ever experienced is filed away in that backpack. So, that pack of yours has a lot of negative stuff inside. But your mind is different. Your mind is like your software—intelligent and up-to-date. It can believe, hope, make decisions, evaluate a situation, and be curious."

He looked up. "So, it's sort of like my brain is on autopilot, and my mind is the pilot."

"Yep. That's exactly right."

When Tyler learned to separate his mind from his brain, profound things started to happen. Suddenly his enemy was cut off at the knees. He became an active creator in his thinking, rather than a passive recipient of its negativity.

When his brain said, "You don't have to start your homework today; you can do it tomorrow," he used his mind to make a different choice: "It's important to get going on my homework. Otherwise, I'll get behind."

When he heard, "You're stupid," he used his mind to turn the negative into something more constructive: "You're not stupid; you're actually pretty smart—sometimes you get things wrong, but most of the time, you do a good job."

Through repetition and practice, he used the power of his mind to overwrite his negative programming. Instead of believing he was dumb and inadequate, he started to see himself as smart and capable. Rather than procrastinating and dragging his feet, he learned to prioritize and stick with his school work. Gradually, he changed his brain from a negative, self-sabotaging monster into a positive, motivated machine of success.

THE SECRET TO TYLER'S SUCCESS

The first critical step Tyler took was to start his journey with a clear vision: "I want to burn my backpack." This goal was crystal clear to him, and he held to it even when the terrain got rocky. Many times he felt like quitting, muttering under his breath, "When am I going to learn to be less afraid? My stupid brain is so stuck." Regardless of setbacks, he stayed in the game and kept his end goal in mind. By devoting himself to therapy, he learned to identify his negative thinking and replace his fears with a more positive mind-set.

The second critical step he took was to learn one of the most important skills in the area of behavioral change—separating the mind from the brain. By recognizing that his brain was the source of his negative thinking and sabotaging behavior, he could use his mind to teach his brain something different. He learned that his brain is a physical organ—a storage container of sensory experiences, both positive and negative. And his mind is the psychological organ—intelligent, savvy, and capable of overwriting negative programming.

Knowing that his mind—and not his "stupid brain"—was in charge of his thinking changed his life forever.

The third critical step he took was to assemble his own support team. After a lengthy self-appointed exile to his dorm room, he had some work to do in this area. His humility and courage allowed him to reach out to others and ask for help. He created a short list of loyal friends and family who could be supportive and hold him accountable to his goals. He made a list of his top three fears, along with action steps and timelines for completion, and circulated it among his support team. Begrudgingly, he joined a community group for depressed teens, and, after the second week, had become fast friends with group members.

At nineteen, Tyler was the poster child of depression, defeat, and pessimism. Two years later, he remains an honor student, is back to being the life of the party, and continues to make a daily to-do list keeping his procrastination at bay.

It's safe to say he really did burn his backpack.

This story demonstrates that change is possible for any of us. By taking three critical steps—creating a vision, mind over matter, and developing a support team—you can change a bad habit into a healthier one.

YOUR BRAIN REALLY CAN CHANGE

Only a few decades ago, scientists considered the human brain something that was fixed, or hardwired. In other words, our brains were believed to have an irreversible quality about them—sort of like a handprint that dries in concrete. Experts assumed that whatever you learned as a young child—overeating, watching TV, inactivity, or avoiding conflict—would stay with you into adulthood. Now, that would really suck. Who wants to be doomed—stuck with bad habits like white on rice? Some refer to this as neurological nihilism—a fancy way of saying your brain won't let you change your bad habits. That's enough to make most of us stay on the couch with the family pack of chips! Why even attempt to swim against the current if you're never going to get anywhere, right?

But hold on . . . this is where it's not so sucky! We're all lucky the neuroplasticians (these are the really smart gals and guys who study the brain) didn't stop here. They continued climbing up the mountain, against many odds, performing hundreds of studies on the brain, only to deliver some of the best news of the twenty-first century. Our brains can change! In fact, they can change dramatically. We can teach our brains to see again (some blindness isn't permanent) and walk (paralysis can be temporary). People who have experienced horrible psychological traumas can reverse their nightmares and fears—hoarders learn to stop stockpiling—and people addicted to chemicals can quit poisoning their bodies. We aren't predestined to repeat the same old habits over and over again. Our brains have what's called neuroplasticity.[1] This just means they are "plastic" and fluid, with the capacity to change and adapt. Instead of the brain being stuck like concrete, it's a living and breathing organism—ever learning, adapting, growing, and expanding.

But here's the rub. Learning a new behavior doesn't happen overnight. Think about it. Have you ever tried to learn a new language, learn to play the piano, or get more organized? It takes recitation and determination to get there. By introducing new habits slowly and consistently, your brain does learn to adapt and change. Pretty soon, you're speaking Spanish, playing Beethoven, and staying organized. It's only because your brain is remembering what you're teaching it. The same holds true for unlearning bad habits. Over time, you can reduce your brain's appetite for cigarettes, alcohol, fatty foods, sugar, TV, and staying glued to the couch.

THE MAGIC BULLET: THREE STEPS TO MAKING A CHANGE

First, you must begin your journey with an act of vision. Start with the end in mind by asking, "What do I really want, and why do I want it?"[2] Visualize your success by imagining yourself at the finish line. Create concrete goals, actions, and timelines for completion.

The starting line for most of us is an epiphany or a groundbreaking emotional experience. The really crappy stuff can kick us into action: Terminal or chronic illness, poor health, or the possibility of losing a valued relationship are the biggies. They are the worst kind of alarm clocks, but they do tend to wake us up and get us motivated to change. But maybe you've just had a good talk with yourself; maybe you realized you're not quite where you want to be. Or maybe you couldn't catch your three-year-old as she ran toward the wall with paint-splattered hands. Maybe it's a class reunion or an upcoming vacation. Regardless, you want to change. You're at the starting line.

Second, it's important to develop the right skills. Successful change has more to do with skill power than will power. In order to change your bad habits into healthier ones, you'll want to learn these five skills, which will be discussed in further detail in the coming chapters:

- Learn about your brain. When changing behavior, your brain can be your greatest ally or the devil on your shoulder. Use your mind to guide your brain by applying "mind over matter" to everyday thoughts, feelings, and behaviors.
- Move a muscle; move a feeling. Learn to use physical movement to address your psychological and emotional barriers.
- Identify perfectionistic tendencies, and reduce their impact on your behavior.
- Stop procrastinating, and start getting results.
- Improve your self-control and your ability to delay gratification.

For the third and final step, you will need to develop the right support team. Bad habits and good habits are almost always socially influenced. To reach your goals, you will need to create a strong network of friends, family, and community support.

The bottom line? Changing behavior can suck. The good news is that with a solid vision, the right skills, and a support network, you can navigate through the sucky waters.

These next few chapters will get you moving in the direction you want to go. You'll move from relying on your pesky brain (hint: it's all about mind over matter) to developing skills like the ability to delay gratification and to curtail perfectionism. You'll wrap things up by getting the right support team on your side.

BEGIN WITH THE END IN MIND

(with thanks to Stephen Covey)

How do you feel when you plan a vacation? If you're like me, you stay inspired because you imagine being on the beach or lounging by the fire at your favorite ski resort. Rather than focusing on the details of getting there— packing, standing at the airport, waiting for a rental car, or even finishing all the work that's at hand before you leave— isn't the vision of that beach or ski resort enough to really get you there? Most of us are pretty successful at vacationing because our minds are imagining how great it will be. Funny, we don't seem to mind the inconvenience that precedes it. In fact, we are determined, committed, and single-minded to just get there.

In the same way, imagining your success is a great way to embark on a new goal. By connecting to who you are becoming and where you are going, you train your mind to think like someone who has already reached his or her destination.

Beginning your journey up the mountain requires three critical steps: unlocking the power of your imagination, creating your vision statement, and setting your goals.

STEP ONE: UNLOCKING THE POWER OF YOUR IMAGINATION

Start by asking yourself several questions. For example, who do you want to be when you grow up? (Yes, even adults can ask this.) What inspires you? Who inspires you, and why? Where do you want to go in life? This is the brainstorming part of your journey where anything and everything is considered. Imagining and dreaming keep you moving your mind before you move your feet.

Think about it this way: You are the CEO of your life. The first thing you need to do is call forth your dream. You can't open the doors of a company (or your life) until you know why your company exists and what it's going to do. In your haste to get results, you can be tempted to skip this critical part of your journey. Setting goals before you create your dream is premature, and arguably one of the biggest barriers to behavioral change. When the climb gets grueling, if your goals aren't linked to your dream, you will lose momentum.

TIP: Dream first, and take action second!

Why Is Your Imagination Critical to Success?

The experts tell us that our subconscious mind can't tell the difference between a real experience and one that is vividly imagined.[1] If you close your eyes and imagine anything—your child's face, a favorite painting, or the letter A—your brain lights up inside as if you were experiencing the real deal.[2] In other words, anything you visualize to be true about yourself is essentially accepted as real by your mind.

If you imagine weighing less, eating healthy, feeling better, and being active, your mind accepts this as your new reality. Now, let's consider the reverse, because it's true there, too: If you think about how hard it will be to go to the gym, or how inconvenient it is to eat healthy food, then you stay stuck—a perpetual cycle of choosing the same old bad habits. Focusing on the negative stuff really slows you down. As great as your imagination is, it can sabotage your goals if you aren't careful. You have to point your imagination in the direction you need it to go.

The Secret to Capturing Your Imagination

Many of us live fast-paced lives with barely enough time left over to clean out the refrigerator—let alone dream about the future. The treadmill of life can keep us from one of the most beautiful and inspiring experiences of being a human being—the ability to dream.

If you're reading this book, you probably want something to be different about your life. In quiet moments, you've probably imagined how your life would be if . . .

. . . if you lost weight, took better care of your body, changed your negative thinking, or stopped procrastinating. We all have our own list of "ifs"—the things we dream about changing, but can't seem to make happen. With a little effort and skill power on your part, you can learn to unlock your dreams and make them a reality.

First, pick something that you love to do—riding a bike, walking through the woods, playing golf, or spending time with your kids. While your mind is relaxed, allow yourself to dream about what you really want from your life. Ask yourself the million-dollar question (or questions): Who do I want to be when I grow up? What really inspires me? What is on my bucket list? What's working in my life? What's not?

TIP: Don't stay stuck in your "if"!

Next, write down your answers in a journal.
Pay attention to everything you're feeling and
thinking, even if it seems insignificant in the
moment. What's most important here is not to
edit your answers. Write down everything—the

TIP: Your dreams
are hidden in the
details.

more, the better. Spend about fifteen minutes a day with
your journal. Do this for fourteen days in a row. After day 14,
read through your entire journal, and underline any
thought, feeling, or idea that seems particularly compelling
to you. You might notice a pattern in what you've written.
(Anything repeated several times is worth noting.) Write
down the top three themes from your journal entries, and
use these to construct your dream.

For example, you might notice that you repeatedly write
about feeling tired, achy, and out of shape. Your dream could
be to improve your physical fitness and live in a body that
feels good.

STEP TWO: CREATE YOUR VISION STATEMENT

The second critical step you need to take is to create a clear
vision statement. You've called forth your dream; now it's
time to decide on a destination. You might dream about living
in the mountains, but at some point, you must decide which
mountain. Your vision statement is a navigational tool that
points you in the right direction (where am I going?) and
functions as a vehicle of inspiration (why am I going there?).

Without a solid vision, you will go nowhere fast—spinning
your wheels and chasing your tail. A vision statement
should include the where and the why.

Here is an example vision statement: "I value my physical
and emotional health, and I want to live a long and full life.

TIP: Live your vision for twenty-four hours. This is where a little investment on your part will pay dividends. Try this: Spend one day with someone whose lifestyle is a healthy one that you think could work for you. Take mental notes. How are this person's choices the same as yours, and how do they differ? If you don't know someone whose lifestyle is one you want to emulate, think more about what you want to change in your own life. Looking to healthy role models can help you get on track.

My final destination is to create a healthy body and mind. I want to think positive and constructive thoughts about myself and feel better in my body physically. I want to be a great role model to my children in this area by taking daily action to improve myself."

Next, create your vision photo. We take photos while on vacation for one reason: We want to remember the moment. The same holds true when you are setting your goals. Imagining yourself at the finish line, in full detail, will keep your vision alive. Remember, anything you imagine about yourself is accepted as real by your mind.

For example, if your goal is to lose a solid twenty pounds, visualize yourself already twenty pounds lighter. How do you feel? Are you more confident, happy? How do people respond to your success? Imagine less back pain, more flexibility, and waking up well rested. If you close your eyes and imagine yourself twenty pounds lighter, your mind will start to accept this as your new reality.

Then, create your vision board. This is a personal favorite, and something I do when setting new goals. Here's how this works: Take a bulletin board, and attach your vision statement and goals. Add items that inspire, such as photos and favorite quotes. Reference it daily. Don't let this out of your sight—keep it front and center at home and the office (you might consider making two boards).

STEP THREE: SET YOUR GOALS

The third critical step is to set your goals. Your goals are what turn your vision into a reality.

A way to start is by taking a written inventory of your habits. Keeping a journal of your fitness and eating behaviors for seven days is a great way to concretely realize just where you are in your fitness and eating habits. Once you've done this, plan a date with yourself to really look at your notes. It should be pretty clear as to what you want to change. Once you pinpoint that, you can create clear goals for yourself, whether it be "lose five pounds" or "limit fast-food meals to one time per week" or "walk fifteen minutes a day for a week, and increase to twenty minutes" or something larger.

Next, start rehearsing the steps you need to take to meet your goals. The experts call this mental practice or mental rehearsing.[3] By imagining your moves ahead of time, you create a magical game of mental chess. You rehearse—in your mind—all of the necessary steps to reaching your goals.

TIP: Keep your goals simple and measurable.

Congratulations! You've just taken your first big step up the mountain—calling forth your dream, creating your vision statement, and setting your goals.

Now, let's keep climbing.

TIP: List the top ten steps you need to take to reach your goals. Here are a few examples:

- Going to the grocery store rather than eating out
- Buying healthy food
- Ordering low-fat options from the menu
- Going to bed earlier so you can get to the gym; keeping your gym bag packed ahead of time
- Walking outside over your lunch hour
- Bringing your lunch to work
- Avoiding the vending machines and the plethora of snack options in the cafeteria.

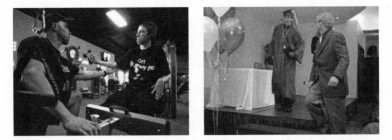

ABOVE LEFT: Daniel and his personal trainer, Doug, at the gym. ABOVE RIGHT: Daniel receiving his high school diploma. Courtesy of the *St. Petersburg Times.*

Get Inspired: Daniel Lowe's Story

DANIEL'S MESSAGE: *Nothing is impossible if you dream big and believe in yourself.*

I was born with cerebral palsy and weighed just two pounds, six ounces, at birth—but I'm told I was quite feisty and breathing without a ventilator within forty-eight hours of arriving. When I was six, I scratched and clawed at the doctors as they cut into my balled-up leg muscles and tendons and put my legs in casts. At seven, I walked for the first time on my own, but tripped and severed an artery.

As I grew, my left foot dragged and my crooked posture got worse. At eighteen, I set a goal to walk across the stage at my high school graduation for my diploma. So I had my hip broken and fastened with six pins. I screamed in pain as nurses bent my knees to my chest during recovery.

After surgery, I lost some of my drive and was depressed. I started skipping school and sleeping longer. My mom thought going to a gym would help, so I started working with a personal trainer at Anytime Fitness. Doug Patton was so determined to help me that he trained me for free.

On my first day, as I sat against a weight bench, my pulse began to race: I was having a seizure and passed out. But I didn't let this stop me and returned to the gym two days later and did cable presses and shoulder lifts and curls. As graduation approached, I went from three sessions a week to four.

When the big day came, I was nervous and my heart was beating fast. What if I tripped? What if the tassel got in my eyes? What if I couldn't grab the diploma? Adrenaline kicked in as I headed toward the stairs. Doug was ready to help, but I wanted to do it on my own. I made it onto the stage, took a couple of steps, grabbed my diploma, traded a handshake, and smiled. Everyone cheered and yelled my name.

When it was over, I took the largest sigh of relief I've ever taken in my life and proclaimed, "I'm a free man." For all the setbacks, pain, and struggle, it was all worth it to claim what was rightfully mine, and to do so on my own two feet.

"This kid *chose* to have his hip broken so he could walk across the stage to pick up his diploma, and you can't get out of bed at 6 am?" —Chuck

MIND OVER MATTER

This next step might be your biggest challenge. If you know anything about mountaineering, then you've heard of the Hillary Step. For climbers to reach the summit of Everest, they must cross a forty-foot spur of snow and ice. Even the most experienced athletes struggle at this section of the mountain. In any endeavor, there is always a point that separates the men from the boys (or the women from the girls). The same is true in the area of behavioral change.

Traversing this section of the mountain requires two critical skills:

1. Understanding how your brain reacts to change (Hint: Your brain doesn't like it.)
2. Applying mind over matter to replace negative thinking with a more positive mind-set.

THE DARK SIDE OF YOUR BRAIN
When you're hoping to change bad habits into good ones, you must understand the brain and how it responds to change, especially when you're thinking about getting healthy and staying healthy.

When you introduce a new behavior such as eating healthier, cutting back on sugar, or increasing your exercise, your brain will be resistant—at least initially. It will complain and create excuses. At times, it will be downright stubborn, refusing to budge. You might start to slip on the ice, fall on the rocks, and fear that you're headed for the nearest crevice (never to be seen again).

During the initial stages of change, your brain is more of an adversary than a friend. It's saying, "Stop doing what you're doing; this doesn't feel comfortable!" In fact, your brain is wired to protect any behavior it is familiar with, even if this habit is destructive to your health.[1]

SOMETIMES OUR BRAINS SABOTAGE US

Let's take smoking—it's a great example here. We all know smoking is unhealthy, but the minute nicotine levels drop, the brain signals a warning bell requesting another cigarette. You can just hear the brain singing its favorite tune, "Baby, come back! You can blame it all on me!"

Why does your brain do this? Changing any habitual behavior will most likely upset the apple cart, scramble the wires, and generally make the brain a bit crabby. In the beginning stages of change, your brain has put out the "Do Not Disturb" sign. At first, eating more vegetables and cutting back on processed food will feel unfamiliar to your brain. Your brain is screaming, "Show me the Pringles!"

And here's why: The brain is trained to see any current behavior as necessary for your survival. Through repetition and habit, you've trained your brain that this particular habit is the right one for your survival. Being sedentary, eating fast food, or clamming up instead of being assertive are all behaviors your brain gets comfortable with and will do almost anything to protect. Once you try altering these behaviors, your brain becomes like a toddler smack in the middle of the terrible twos, stomping around and yelling, "No, I don't want to, and you can't make me!"

Just because your brain can get you through college doesn't mean this organ is the smartest thing on the planet. In fact, your brain can be downright thick-skinned, obsessive, demanding, and shortsighted; it can turn into the ultimate excuse-making machine. Think of the cartoon devil on your shoulder, the greatest of all seducers.

When you give in by eating the doughnut, staying on the couch, or overspending, you feel temporarily comforted. Your brain says, "Ah, this feels good! Thank you."

Temporary comfort is just that, temporary. It doesn't get you where you need to go in life, and it doesn't serve your greater vision to live a healthier life.

I've been there. The other guys writing this book? Chuck's been there, Brian's been there. All of our Anytime Fitness clients? Been there. You've been there, too.

ROCKY TERRAIN AHEAD

Even though your brain isn't hardwired for life, it's resistant to change. We all have our own psychological blueprint, a mental image of how we think about ourselves, and this directs how we navigate through life.[2] Did you know that your blueprint is formed by the time you are five years old? Doesn't seem fair, but most of us learned some pretty negative stuff before we learned to put on mascara or drive a car. Your blueprint got started from other people's opinions and treatment of you. If you receive negative messages about yourself, that's what you start to believe. "Garbage in, garbage out," applies here. Your negative, self-sabotaging thinking has been around for a long time. It's very old—and stubborn.

Here are a few examples of negative blueprints: Do any of these sound familiar?

- I'm stupid and inadequate.
- I don't want to start exercising—it's too hard.
- I can't ever seem to finish anything I start.
- I'm unworthy of success.
- I'm not capable of success.
- I need to be in control of everything in order to be successful.
- I will always be fat.
- I just don't have what it takes—I'm going to fail.
- I have to be perfect; I can't make any mistakes.
- I'm responsible for other people's thoughts, feelings, and behavior.
- Other people's opinion of me matters more to me than my own.

Negative thinking patterns keep you afraid, anxious, guilty, and depressed. And, surprise, surprise, your behavior follows: You might procrastinate, blow up at people, avoid conflict, try to control everything, or get caught up in the details, losing sight of the big picture. Negative thoughts sabotage your goals, sending you down a one-way road of fear, avoidance, and underperformance. When you're thinking in more positive ways, your behavior will be more constructive. You'll be likely to stay focused, be direct and honest in your communication, and retain the optimism needed to prevail against obstacles.

Okay, I can hear you thinking, "Easy for you to say, but is it really possible to change the soundtrack?"

A WHOLE NEW MIND-SET: MAKING IT OVER THE HILLARY STEP
The most challenging part of your climb will be to transform your brain from a sabotaging bully into a goal-achieving friend. To do this, you will need to learn the most important skill in behavioral change—separating your mind from your brain.

Quick reminder: The brain is a physical organ and the source of your negative thinking and sabotaging behavior. It's a storage container of every single one of your experiences—both positive and negative (an outdated hard drive playing on repeat). But, your mind is different. It's a psychological organ with intelligent and up-to-date software. Your mind can believe, hope, make decisions, evaluate a situation, and be curious. It's the primary vehicle to overwriting your negative thinking.

Here is how you use your mind to traverse a forty-foot spur of snow and ice—in five easy steps!

1. Identify your negative thinking. Write down your negative thoughts word for word in your journal. You will notice that certain thoughts repeat themselves over and over. We all have our own negative tapes that love to play on repeat. (Refer to the list in "Rocky Terrain Ahead," above, for examples.)

2. What are your triggers? A trigger is something that prompts your negative thinking. These are very individualized; what triggers one person may not trigger somebody else. To identify your own triggers, you'll need to pay attention to what's going on when your brain starts getting negative. Some examples are negative feedback from others, distraction and overstimulation, the lack of feeling supported or validated, a

disorganized work space, and failure to complete a project on time. Sometimes our negative thoughts surface when we are surrounded by unhealthy distractions—TV, junk food, and negative people.

3. Use your mind to craft a positive and constructive statement to challenge each negative thought. Write this down in your journal. For example, if your brain says, "I can start exercising tomorrow," use your mind to create a new thought: "It would be healthier for me to start my good habits today. If I start small—all I have to do right now is walk for fifteen minutes—tomorrow, I can increase it to twenty."

4. Mentally rehearse your positive thoughts daily. It takes repetition to change your brain's wiring. Refer to your journal daily, and keep practicing.

5. Trust your goals and your vision, not your brain! During the initial stages of change, your goals are more trustworthy than your brain. When your brain gets cranky and resistant, just keep climbing. Keep sight of your goals—don't lose your footing.

THE 66-DAY RULE

Phillippa Lally and her colleagues at University College London have made some remarkable observations about how people succeed in developing good habits.[3] These researchers found that for most people, it takes roughly 66 days for a good habit to become ingrained. Before you start thinking, "Wait, what about this 21-day stuff?" hang with me: After about 21 days, your brain starts to develop muscle memory for your new thinking and habits. This is when your brain starts remembering your new behavior. It's thinking, "Oh, I know what you're doing, and I'm feeling more comfortable with this new habit." So, the first 21 days are pretty important to form new habits.

At about day 66, Lally observed, your brain does something pretty amazing. It starts to adopt your new habit as the one it wants to keep. Think about it like this: Days 1 through 21 are sort of like the dating phase for your brain. Although it's trying on the new habit, it may not be sold on the change. During the first 21 days, your brain is still a bit undecided as to whether it wants to get rid of your old habit and keep the new one, but these days are still crucial for getting the new habits in place. Days 22 through 66 are the engagement phase. Your brain is more committed and is thinking, "I want to marry this habit. I'm sold that this is the one for me."

The bottom line is this: These 66-day plans are immensely successful. They are a critical starting point in behavioral change. You'll want to make sure to give yourself plenty of time to learn and grow into your new habit. Sixty-six days might feel like an enormous chunk of time. So, the best way to get moving is to break it up into smaller chunks. This is why the 21-day plan is so critical. Start with a 21-day plan. Then gradually increase to 30 days, then 40, and so on. (For some concrete 21-day plans, check out the nutrition and fitness chapters).

Get Inspired: Susan Bock's Story

SUSAN'S MESSAGE: *Loving yourself and realizing that you are worth the effort is the first step toward a better life.*

Virtually my entire life, I have struggled with my weight. As a fat little girl, I was made fun of a lot and would often come

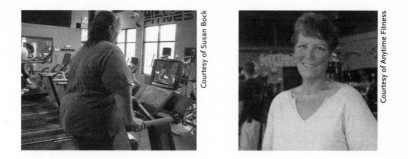

Courtesy of Susan Bock

Courtesy of Anytime Fitness

home from school crying. I wasn't sure if I had a place in this world.

Over the years, I tried almost every fad diet, only to end up weighing more than when I started. In 1978, I had gastric bypass surgery. When it failed, I concluded that I was destined to remain fat. I began to drink heavily in order to numb the pain.

At age forty-nine, I was at my heaviest—450 pounds and suffering from high blood pressure, joint pain, sciatica, and depression. I remember falling in my bedroom and spending an hour trying to figure out how to get up. I had this horrible fear of something like that happening while I was in public.

One day, while watching a popular weight-loss TV program, I realized that exercising was the one thing I had never tried to do to lose weight. I guess I just always thought I was too big—but when I saw people who looked just like me doing it, I thought maybe I could, too.

I finally began turning my life around with the help of a personal trainer at my local Anytime Fitness gym. In just a few short months, I lost 75 pounds! To date, I have lost just over 200 pounds. I'm doing all the things I never thought I could—hiking, running, riding a bike.

I am living proof that struggles can be overcome through sacrifice, perseverance, and patience. I have finally learned what living your life is, compared with just existing in life. And, there's no better feeling.

"I've known Susan for a few years and have noticed that her physical appearance isn't her most notable change. She's happier, more confident and smiles more often—and fills herself with soul calories every day."
—Chuck Runyon

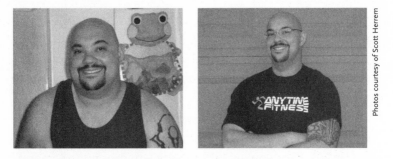

Photos courtesy of Scott Herrem

Get Inspired: Scott Herrem's Story

SCOTT'S MESSAGE: *There's nothing wrong with setting the bar high. You can do anything you set your mind to.*

The beginning of 2008 is when I decided to change my life. After seeing myself in the mirror at a bloated 320-plus pounds, a pack-a-day smoker, with no energy to play with my daughter or fulfill my duties as a deputy sheriff, I knew I wasn't the man I wanted to be. As a former athlete, I knew that my mental state was crushed under the weight of my physical condition.

I had the desire to change, but felt overwhelmed about where to begin or where to go to get in shape. A friend of mine brought me to his Anytime Fitness gym, and my weight loss began to take off. I quickly learned that this wasn't a gym for the superbuff or the "beautiful people." This truly was a gym for all people and all fitness levels. With diet and nutritional support from my wife, Katie, all that was left was to work off the pounds.

Steadily, I lost 113 pounds and was featured in a local coupon ad, which gave me more motivation to work even harder. More importantly, my daughter noticed my hard work and was proud of her "skinny daddy." The manager at my club was always kind and recognized all the hard work I put in, and he nominated me for a national Anytime Fitness award. In 2009, I was selected as an Anytime Fitness national success story. The experience was amazing. A video chronicling my journey, which now airs on the Internet, keeps me humble and reminds me of where I came from.

Most amazing to me is the response I received from other people, both in my community and across the country. Once, while I was on duty as a deputy sheriff, someone called our dispatch from New Jersey and asked to speak to the "Anytime Fitness Deputy." He was in a situation similar to mine when I began my weight loss and wanted to tell me that my story inspired him to take action. Several other people have contacted me via Facebook to tell me how much they relate to my story.

I'm incredibly proud to say that my mom, wife, and fellow deputies have joined me in making healthy living a priority.

Today, with every drop of sweat that I rinse from myself, I get back a little piece of the man I once lost.

"Once Scott saved his own life, he put himself in a better position to save others." —Chuck Runyon

MOVE A MUSCLE,
MOVE A FEELING

If you've ever sat across from Chuck Runyon, then you know something about "Move a muscle, move a feeling." After about ten minutes in the same position, he starts to fidget. It starts in his jaw, moves down to his shoulders, and eventually lands in his legs. At this point, he usually stands up, picks up his golf club, and starts swinging at an imaginary ball.

At first I thought this was a mild case of attention deficit, but upon closer observation, I realized that something else was going on with Chuck.

So, I finally asked, "Why do you move around so much in meetings? Seems like it's hard for you to sit still—just curious."

Without missing a beat, he said, "My mind works better when I'm moving around. If I get up and start moving, I can think clearly—more creatively."

Physical movement connects Chuck to his creative edge. By moving his body, his brain fires up (his neurons start dancing around) and he's ready to respond to just about anything you can throw at him.

And, Chuck is not the only one who understand this. Just recently, I met David, a fifteen-year-old who couldn't learn algebra. He was really down in the dumps about his struggles to complete his homework.

He looked at me with total frustration. "I just don't get it," he said. "I'm sitting at my desk, staring at my algebra book, and nothing seems to be happening. I'm really trying to figure this stuff out, but I just can't get it."

Remembering Chuck's strategy, I asked, "Well, how long do you sit at that desk of yours?"

TIP: When your brain gets stuck—move your body!

"I don't know . . . probably a whole hour. And nothing happens—nothing. It's like my mind is just blank."

"David, have you ever tried getting out of that darn chair and walking around your room instead of staring at your book?"

He nodded. "I have thought about that. But I thought I was supposed to stay in the chair."

"Well, maybe you don't have to."

He smiled. "That sounds good," he said. (This is a fifteen-year-old's dream—not having to sit still. Teenagers hate sitting, and there's a reason for this).

"Try walking around when you're reading your homework, or at least take some breaks—maybe every ten minutes or so—get up and move around."

"How's that gonna help?"

"Moving your body will help your brain think better. If you start moving, your brain will follow."

Two days later, I got a call from a very happy mom. "David finished his homework last night," she said. "Can you believe it? He was doing the strangest thing—moving and pacing the whole time."

THE POWER OF PHYSICAL MOVEMENT:
TEN SECONDS IS ALL IT TAKES

One of the most compelling aspects of our brain is that it learns in multiple ways. We've mostly been talking about the thinking aspect of your brain—using your mind to tell your brain something new. Thinking happens inside your head—it is an intellectual process and has its inherent limitations. We all know about writer's block or brain freezes, when your brain is essentially stuck in one place (usually negative) and doesn't want to budge. You might be caught in a cycle of procrastination, chronic worry, or pessimistic thinking. Maybe you're stuck in feelings of sadness, fear, insecurity, or resentment. Regardless of what you say to yourself, you're unable to change your negative thoughts and feelings.

Think about Chuck and David. Physical movement helps their brains stay active, positive, and creative. When they feel a brain block coming on, they get up and start moving around. Ten seconds of physical movement can begin to transform a negative thought into something more positive and a negative feeling into something more pleasurable and optimistic. Moving your body can instantly shift your mind-set.

Consider a very simple example. If you're stuck in negative thinking ("I don't want to work out today—the couch feels way too comfortable and working out is hard"; "Who cares if I eat the entire pizza?" or "I'll always be overweight"), try moving your body as a way to shift your thinking. Get off the couch and out of your chair—and start moving. Walk around for a few minutes. Notice what happens to your mind.

Once you start moving around even a little bit, you might start thinking, "Working out does suck at times, but all I need to do right now is walk for fifteen minutes." Or "It does matter if I eat a whole pizza by myself—maybe, one piece is all I need." Or "I am feeling sluggish and tired, but walking around is starting to make me feel more positive things— I'm feeling a bit more energized, less cranky, and more motivated."

Frequent brain locks or cycles of negative thinking can make it almost impossible for you to reach your goals. These cycles are incredibly demotivating and can put you back to square one in an instant. Don't let them. Recognize them and fight back. To reach the top of your mountain, you will want to learn how to stop this self-sabotaging cycle. Follow these steps:

- If you are in a brain lock, or negative thinking cycle, for more than ten minutes (and mind over matter isn't working), stop thinking, and start moving.
- Be proactive. Move your body every hour—sitting for long periods can reduce your motivation and brain-power.
- Build in short walks (three to ten minutes) during your workday (not to the vending machine).
- Identify blocks in your thinking and emotions. Notice when you are stuck in the negative zone, and take immediate action.
- Consider adding physical activity as one of your personal goals: Even ten to fifteen minutes a day can make a difference.

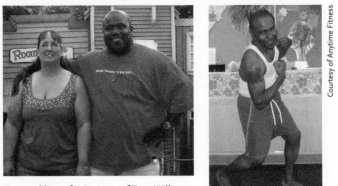

Tony and his wife. Courtesy of Tony Williams.

Get Inspired: Tony Williams's Story

TONY'S MESSAGE: *Take control of your health before it's too late.*

At thirty-seven years old, I was told I would be lucky to live until forty. At five feet five, I was 294 pounds, with hypertension, sleep apnea, and high cholesterol. As a railroad worker, I have unconventional work hours, so it was easy for me to fall into the trap of a sedentary lifestyle that involved eating fast food all the time.

After my doctor revealed the seriousness of my health issues, I decided to join Weight Watchers with my mom and wife. As the weight began dropping, my energy level rose, so I strove to become more active. I played Wii *Fit* and began walking and biking. I also decided to join a local gym, choosing Anytime Fitness because it was open twenty-four hours a day and could cater to my crazy work hours. It was there that I incorporated cardio and strength training into my exercise routine.

Since I began my journey back to good health, I have lost 121 pounds! I now serve as a spokesperson for the railroad and give regular speeches to my fellow railroaders (more than six hundred of them) about the importance of healthy living.

To everyone out there, know that I have no iron will. There is nothing that makes me extraordinary. I don't have Jillian Michaels on speed dial. All I did was utilize the tools at my disposal to improve and extend my life.

"What's more expensive; a heart attack or a gym membership?" —Chuck Runyon

I WOULD KILL FOR CHOCOLATE!

So far, so good. You're setting your goals, you know what your pesky brain is up to, and you're committed to the challenge. Great, from zero to sixty . . . Go!

Not so fast. In the area of behavioral change, one of the biggest obstacles is changing too quickly. In some instances, going cold turkey is the most effective route. But in many cases, our brains will interpret too rapid a change as a stressful event.[1]

Once your brain decides that a new behavior is stressful, it will fight to bring the old behavior back to restore normalcy and balance. This creates a natural barrier to change.

The all-too-famous plan to eliminate all sugar is a great example of when faster can be slower. Sure, you might succeed for a few days, but by day three, you're ready to kill for a bowl of Frosted Mini-Wheats. Your brain is in meltdown, your body is in withdrawal, and you are crabby as all get-out. Really, really crabby. To satisfy the urge, do you eat just one? Nope. Like many of us, you end up making up for lost time by eating the entire box. We've all been there.

Here's the deal: Your brain is a creature of habit; it loves the status quo. Any change will be automatically interpreted as awkward and a threat to your identity—at least at first.

C'mon, isn't changing at lightning speed usually a good thing?

Not when it comes to the brain. Easy does it, slow and steady. Too many changes at once, and you might start sliding down the mountain.

A JOURNEY OF A THOUSAND MILES STARTS WITH ONE STEP

When embarking on a new goal, it can be tempting to try to climb the whole mountain in one day. And we all know what happens when we do that! Slow, steady, and consistent climbing is the most efficient way to reach the summit. Your brain responds favorably to incremental change—change that occurs one step at a time. In fact, any change you make—smoking five cigarettes instead of ten, adding vegetables to your evening meal, or walking ten minutes every day—will start to alter the physical structure of your brain.[2] Although supersized accomplishments are worth pursuing— running a marathon or working out seven days a week—they aren't necessary to living a healthy life.

Here are a few tips to keep you moving forward, rather than sliding downhill.

1. Divide your goals into smaller, digestible steps. To keep things on an even keel, avoid making extreme changes. So instead of saying, "I will never, ever have sugar again" (and pretty much setting yourself up to trip on the rocks), try simply reducing your intake or weeding out sugar from particular meals on a daily basis. Rather than swearing up and down that you'll go to the gym seven days a week, try going every other day or committing to two or three regular days at first.

2. Build in little incentives along the way. Maybe, you pick one day to eat your favorite dessert, get movie popcorn (with butter) on a Saturday night, or treat yourself to a massage with the money you save from not eating out. You stay motivated if you divide your goals into smaller pieces, rather than biting off one big chunk. If you want to lose ten pounds, build in a reward for every two pounds lost. Your brain loves rewards and anything else pleasurable. By adding some fun along the way, you will be more and more likely to continue your climb up the mountain—and that mountain will look less and less like Everest.

3. Take a rest day. Climbing at high altitude requires frequent periods of acclimatization and rest. High-performing athletes are often instructed to take days off—to give their bodies time to soak up the benefits of hard work. If you keep climbing when exhausted and overwhelmed, you'll be likely to start undoing the progress you've made.

Get Inspired: Darren Williams's Story

DARREN'S MESSAGE: *Don't try to hit a home run right away; try some singles first.*

In October 2008, I weighed 452 pounds and was scared to death that my three-year-old daughter would grow up without her father. I can vividly remember thinking that there was a real possibility that I might never get the chance to walk her down the aisle, or play with my grandchildren, or just be there for her.

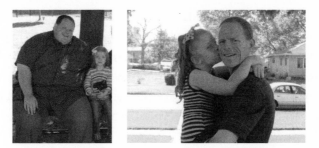

Darren and his daughter. Courtesy of Darren Williams.

I had struggled with my weight my entire life, but 452 pounds was the heaviest I'd ever been. My blood pressure was an elevated 155/95, and I was having severe anxiety attacks about my heart failing. I couldn't live like that anymore. My family deserved better, and so did I.

I began with a walk outside—and it wasn't easy. I was out of breath, and my back and legs ached. Soon, I decided to join the neighborhood Anytime Fitness—it's open twenty-four hours, so now, there really were no more excuses! At the gym, my workout regimen started with my walking at two miles per hour on the treadmill for ten to fifteen minutes.

I took this same do-it-in-moderation approach with portion control. Instead of going from the 4,000 to 5,000 calories I was consuming daily to 1,200 calories—I had tried this in the past and it never worked—I reduced calories gradually, setting goals of where I wanted to be, and tracking my daily

---

TIP: If you become overly stressed with a goal for more than a few days in a row, stop and take one rest day—resume your goal the next day.

---

intake against that goal. I also made changes in the type of food I ate—shifting from fast food and other fatty foods to more home-cooked meals and more vegetables. I used to drink a lot of regular soda and hated the taste of diet soda. I slowly made the switch by allowing myself one regular soda a day, and then eventually made the transition to diet and more water.

Today, I run 6½ to 7 miles per day on the treadmill at 6½ miles per hour. I lift weights three times a week and ride on the stationary bike three or four times a week. My diet consists of between 1,800 and 2,200 calories. I still continue to have treats from time to time—I just have to plan for them and either cut calories other times of the day or work out a little bit harder at the gym.

My transformation didn't happen overnight, and it still takes work every day—but nothing is greater than being able to be here for my daughter, not to mention being fit enough to keep up with her!

"Your daughter or son doesn't care how much you can lift. They only care that you can lift them." —Chuck Runyon

Get Inspired: Jeremy and Susie Bowen's Story

JEREMY AND SUSIE'S MESSAGE: *Put forth the effort, and make time for exercising.*

As working parents catering to our children's busy schedules, we found it hard to exercise and eat right. We were junk-food junkies on a destructive path. It got to the point where we were eating out five days a week: Chips with queso, a Mexican entrée, and dessert. Throw in a few deep-

fried mozzarella sticks for a bedtime snack, and you had an average day of eating for the Bowen
family.

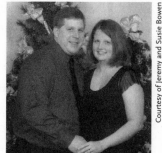

Courtesy of Jeremy and Susie Bowen

Before we knew it, I [Susie]
reached 187 pounds and Jeremy
was nearing 300 pounds. For me,
the wake-up call was stepping on
the scale at the hospital where I
work as a nurse, and thinking,
"Oh, God, I'm thirteen pounds
away from two hundred." And, for
Jeremy it was the realization that
he was on his way to being the
same weight as his dad at 500
pounds.

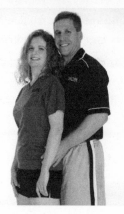

Courtesy of Anytime Fitness

We knew we had to change
course, so we made a pact to join
the local gym and start getting
healthy together.

I started with slow walks on the treadmill and, within a
month, had graduated to tough workouts on the elliptical
machine. Jeremy, who works the swing shift in a steel mill,
would hit the gym late at night because he didn't want to be
seen struggling through his workouts.

"In my head," he said, "I was still the athlete from high
school, so I was very self-conscious about it. I would make
sure no one was there, and go in. Then I could go as hard as
I could and take breaks when I needed to."

We also made some changes in the kitchen: We put away
the fryer, got rid of sugary cereals, and stocked up on
healthy foods. We still eat out, but now it's with a healthy

twist. We used to just look for whatever filled us up most. Now, we're picking places because the grilled chicken is good.

Our new lifestyle has improved our relationship with each other and with our kids. We can now keep up with them, which is something we struggled to do before! We used to say we would grow old and fat together, and now, the only thing that's still true is the growing-old part.

"Underneath the fat, Jeremy and Susan found more love and respect. And I bet they're having more sex." —Chuck Runyon

EVERY MOUNTAINEER STUMBLES: THE MYTH OF PERFECTION

At no time during your ascent will the mountain take a rest day. It will keep giving you one challenge after another—some expected, but most of them surprises. You'll probably slip and stumble all the way to the top. When embarking on a new goal, we all cherish the days when everything is going our way, the sun is out, the weather is perfect, our thinking is positive, and we're feeling motivated and optimistic.

Successful changers understand how to turn a bad day into a better day by making friends with their mistakes and learning to roll with the punches.

Perfectionistic thinking can be one of the biggest obstacles to reaching our health and wellness goals. Perfectionism, also known as dichotomous, or black-and-white, thinking, is common when we are trying to change a behavior. Our brains seem to like this way of thinking, and it can get us in a rut pretty quickly.

Black-and-white thinking promotes extreme behavior. You see yourself as either on a diet or off a diet, as unhealthy or healthy, as good or bad, as succeeding or failing.

Exercise like crazy, or not at all. Watch every single calorie you put in your mouth, or care less about healthy eating.

It's easy to think that an extreme change is the answer. And it is, for a brief moment. Think about those diets that promise extreme weight loss in a matter of days. Sure, you're going to lose weight consuming nothing but hot water, a banana, and cayenne pepper—that's not rocket science. And it's not sustainable. Even changing from four thousand calories a day to a quarter of that . . . better for you, but drastic—and you may be sabotaging yourself.

ANOTHER ROCKY DESCENT

The myth of perfectionism has been around forever and really gets in the way of being healthy. For some of us, perfectionistic thinking is a blueprint we've had since childhood. In fact, the experts now know that we aren't born perfectionists.[1] Over time, we start to internalize other people's expectations of us, losing sight of our own measurement of success.

And it's pretty easy to see how this thinking style sabotages our goals. It creates unrealistic expectations. Instead of striving for excellence, we demand perfection. (Yes, there's a difference between the two.) We might believe we need to have the perfect body, eating habits, and exercise program. We believe we must do it exactly right, or not at all.[2]

Maybe you've created goals that are impossible to reach, and then you get down on yourself when you fail. Trying to lose ten pounds in one week, removing all unhealthy foods, or demanding daily exercise can backfire and really get you in a slump.

Pretty soon, you get negative—really negative. You start avoiding your goals and doubting your abilities. "I'll start tomorrow" becomes the mantra. Instead of focusing on your amazing abilities to learn and adapt, you worry about missing the mark. You become a walking, talking report card—in a constant state of criticism.

Talk about something that sucks! This is the ultimate in self-defeat.

REVISING YOUR THINKING: THE CONTINUUM OF SUCCESS

To be successful in changing unhealthy habits into healthier ones, it is important to look at your life as more of a continuum—not so much perfectionism and failure, but a continuum of success. Some days, you will be closer to success than others.

To avoid going to extremes, think about this: Imagine you're driving and your only goal is to stay within the lines. You might veer a little to the left and then to the right, but your goal is to head for the center. Your car doesn't follow a straight line. No way! It's in a constant state of correction.

Now think about your goals in the same way. For example, if your goal is to work out five days a week, and you miss three days in a row, that's not an invitation to beat yourself up and return to the La-Z-Boy with a supersized pack of Cheetos. Instead, try to think about this as an opportunity to get back on the road. A little patch of gravel doesn't have to push you in the ditch, resigned to total failure.

Successful changers understand that any so-called failure or success is momentary and shouldn't be taken too seriously. If you do miss a workout or fall off your diet, you don't need to beat yourself up. Just pick yourself up, and get back on track.

When planning your goals, think of the 80/20 rule: Stay on track 80 percent of the time, and you will be successful.

To help you—and your brain—think healthy, follow these steps:

Step One: Take inventory of your perfectionistic thinking— do any of these sound familiar?

I'm never good enough.
I'm afraid to start a project for fear it won't be perfect.
Mistakes mean failure.
What other people think of me really matters.
I have to be the best.
I need to hide my mistakes from others.

Step Two: Once you've pinpointed your perfectionistic thinking, strive to create more balanced thinking—remember that continuum—by doing the following:

- Avoid setting extreme goals—divide goals into smaller, digestible steps.
- Keep track of your successes and setbacks in a journal.
- Learn to evaluate your progress toward your goals honestly, by asking yourself, "Am I happy with it?" and "What can I do differently next time?"

Step Three: Make friends with your mistakes. A great way to start doing this is by writing about them in your journal or sharing them with a friend.

Step Four: Reward your effort, rather than the result. Some days are better than others—it's the effort that really matters.

Step Five: Do activities that are pleasurable, as well as challenging.

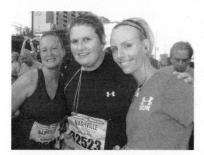

Kendra (at right) celebrates her first half marathon. Courtesy of Kendra Brooks.

Get Inspired: Kendra Brooks's Story

KENDRA'S MESSAGE: *There's no better nourishment than discovering your own inner strength.*

Imagine putting locks on your kitchen cabinets and refrigerator so that you won't binge and purge the food hidden inside. Well, that's what I did for a number of years as I struggled with anorexia and bulimia.

In a last-ditch effort to take control of my own health, I connected with a personal trainer at Anytime Fitness. The trainer helped me incorporate appropriate exercise into my recovery, teaching me how to make my body stronger by working out and developing a new friendly relationship with food.

I started to see definition in my arms and legs and began to slowly increase my strict calorie intake. Vegetables and fruits became a regular part of my diet, and I loved the way they tasted. Why had I cut out green beans from my diet? Why did I not allow myself to eat a tomato? Not only were these foods delicious, but the nutrients made my body feel amazing.

My face began to fill out, my hair had a beautiful shine to it, and my nails were actually starting to grow. I scheduled a physical with my general care physician and passed with flying colors.

It wasn't all a walk in the park, though. I did have my setbacks—especially when people would tell me they were so happy I was gaining weight. When I would hear that, I would revert back to having a negative body image. I even reinstated the locks on my cabinets.

But then I was presented with a challenge—run a half marathon to help raise money for a charity event. Little did I know that this marathon would be a watershed moment in my life. As I ran those thirteen miles, I saw my life come full circle, and I promised myself that when I crossed that finish line, I would leave my eating disorder behind for good. If I could run this half marathon—something I never thought my body would be capable of accomplishing—then I could do anything I set my mind to.

Today, I am more comfortable in my body than I have ever been, and I feel strong physically and mentally. When I walked into the gym, I was 106 pounds. Today, I am 128 pounds and proud of it.

"Physical strength creates mental strength: Kendra outworked and outran her personal demons." —Chuck Runyon

BUT I WANT IT NOW!

Here are perhaps two of the suckiest parts (at least, initially) of changing behavior. Learning to delay gratification and maintain self-control are skills critical to changing a bad habit into a healthier one.

Let's face it. Most of us don't like to wait, for anything. We all have that gimme-gimme-gimme childlike quality that doesn't want to wait to enjoy ourselves. Sitting at a stoplight or standing in line is enough to drive most of us crazy. And these things just take a few minutes. Imagine how impatient we can get when a goal takes weeks or months to complete.

How the heck are we going to change a bad habit if we can't learn to wait?

Wanting to get things now really complicates this whole business of change. We can become disillusioned, expecting great results in the blink of an eye. When that doesn't happen, we have a tendency to throw in the towel.

I've certainly been known to roll my eyes and stomp my feet when I don't get something right away. And I bet I'm not alone there!

Delaying gratification is a form of self-discipline: giving up what you want right now for getting what you want in the future. You won't get to the top of your mountain without this skill.

THE MAGIC BULLET: FIVE CRITICAL STEPS TO DELAYING
GRATIFICATION AND IMPROVING YOUR SELF-CONTROL

The first step is to revisit your vision statement and goals. Keep your eye on the prize—this will give you something positive to focus on when an impulse comes along. Your vision can remind you that your long-term goal is worth some temporary discomfort. You will be less likely to give into distractions.

Second, you need to make sure your vision board, which was discussed earlier in the book and is a physical representation of your vision and inspiration, is visible at work and at home. (This physical symbol of your vision can't help you if it's sitting in the closet.) Visibility is the key. You want it to catch your attention, shift your mind-set, and stimulate positive thoughts. Remember to include your vision statement and goals on your board.

Third, make your environment work for you. You've heard the adage "Keep good things close and convenient, and bad things distant and difficult." Adjust your surroundings to help you think positively about your new habit. Add as many barriers as you can between you and your urges: Keep the peanut butter above your reach, and leave the ice cream at the grocery store. On the flip side, make it easier to do things that are good for you: Keep your gym bag packed, create a workout you can do at home, stock your fridge with healthy food, and bring your lunch to work.

Fourth, keep your goals simple and achievable. You want to feel some challenge on a daily basis, but feeling overwhelmed compromises your self-control. Stress makes you really want stuff like sugar, salt, fat, alcohol, and a long stay on the couch.

The fifth and final step for improving your self-control and ability to accept delayed gratification is to create incentives along the way to keep you feeling good. For example, even if you don't completely meet a goal you have set—and who among us always meets every goal?—allow yourself the gratification of knowing that you did better than you would have, had you not made any effort at all. Giving yourself small rewards along the way will keep you moving in a positive direction. But make sure your rewards don't compromise your goals. Instead of eating the entire tub of ice cream, try enjoying a moderate portion of your favorite dessert every Saturday night.

A few more tips can help you get better at delaying gratification. Try the ones that work for you, or think up new ways.

- For the first thirty days, avoid people and places that remind you of your bad habit.
- Make a game of your goals. Include family and friends for some fun competition. Who can save the most money in one month? Who can eat the most vegetables in one week? And so on.
- If you have an impulse, wait it out for thirty minutes before indulging. Think about what giving in to the urge would mean: Will the fleeting joy of that doughnut really be worth it?

Congrats! You've established your goals, applied mind over matter, and learned some important mountaineering skills. Now, let's talk about the final step you need to take— assembling your team.

Get Inspired:
Chastidy Liebi's Story

CHASTIDY'S MESSAGE: *If you have time to watch TV, then you have time to work out. Don't put it off any longer!*

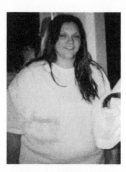

When I gave birth to my second child at twenty-two, I weighed 308 pounds. I was ashamed to be seen in public and had no energy to play with my kids. My doctor told me I was at risk for many diseases related to obesity, including heart disease and diabetes.

Joining a gym wasn't an easy thing for me to do. I was scared! I had never really been in a gym before, and I thought gyms were only for extremely fit people. I felt as if I didn't belong and as if everyone would be judging me. I decided my fears of being uncomfortable weren't worth risking my health and even possibly my life, so I joined Anytime Fitness in Jefferson City, Missouri.

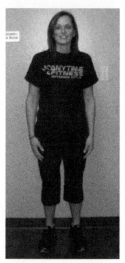

ABOVE: Chastidy, March 2010. BELOW: Chastidy, March 2011. Courtesy of Chastidy Liebi.

I hired a personal trainer and remember being too lazy to keep up during those first few sessions. I wanted to quit, but when I didn't, I felt as if I accomplished something, and it kept me motivated to keep going. I used to struggle walking up the stairs or going to get the mail, but once I started working out, I found energy I didn't know existed. Since joining the gym in May 2010, I have lost more than 150 pounds and just completed my first marathon.

If I could offer any advice, it would be that this is a lifestyle change, not a temporary diet. It takes a lot of hard work and dedication not only from yourself but also from friends and family. The weight wasn't put on overnight, so you can't expect it to come off right away, either.

"From muffin top to MILF, this young lady changed her life and more importantly, the lives of her kids. Never mess with a determined Mom."
—Chuck Runyon

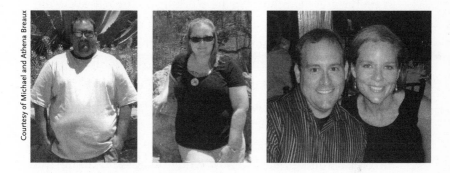

Courtesy of Michael and Athena Breaux

Get Inspired: Michael and Athena Breaux's Story

MICHAEL AND ATHENA'S MESSAGE: *Develop a no-more-excuses mantra. If you truly want to change, then you can—and will—find the time.*

After years of going up and down on the scale, we decided to get serious about our health. The turning point for us was when Michael began having chest pains at thirty-three years old. Michael was also taking blood pressure medication and was diagnosed with sleep apnea. It was time to get back in control of our lives.

NBC's program *The Biggest Loser* was a huge motivator—seeing people with similar conditions winning their personal weight-loss battles. We began by reducing our caloric intake and saw results, which motivated us to keep going. When we decided to get professional help to learn about exercise, we joined an Anytime Fitness club in Eunice, Louisiana, and signed up for sessions with a personal trainer. We learned about proper weight training and cardiovascular fitness. Over time, to our surprise, we actually came to enjoy going to the gym. Funny how we used to say we didn't have the time to exercise! A year later, we are working out nearly every day.

Despite still having to battle our food demons every day, we now have more energy and feel the best we've felt in our lives. We realize that the initial weight loss fed into our desire to challenge ourselves physically. This physical activity helped us build and maintain the healthy lifestyle changes that led to greater weight loss.

Today, the world has opened up to us in ways we could never have imagined. We now enjoy biking and hiking and are looking forward to traveling. We've always dreamed of going to Europe, but didn't want to be seen as the "fat Americans." With a trip planned for Italy and Greece, we cannot wait to get out and experience all that life has to offer.

"From walking on the treadmill to walking through the streets of Greece, exercise is your ticket to living at full capacity. You can't see the world if you can't see your feet." —Chuck Runyon

STRENGTH IN NUMBERS

Here's something that doesn't suck: the buddy system. Climbing any mountain requires a team of solid, loyal support. Did you know that by combining individual discipline with outside support, you improve your odds of meeting any goal?[1] Say you've always wanted to run a nine-minute mile; research has shown that you will reach this goal faster if you join a running club, hire a trainer, or start blogging. (Yes, despite our impending iDeath, even technology can help be a support system).

Successful changers understand the intrinsic value of social influence and support. Whether they are starting a weight loss program, training for a marathon, or modifying their diet, they know their performance will greatly improve with support from family, friends, and the community.

CLIMBING A MOUNTAIN ALONE SUCKS!

As you know, changing old habits into healthier ones creates stress on your brain and your current way of doing life. It can make you slip on the rocks and fall on the ice. Having support available is a protective factor during times of change, making it less likely to abandon our goals when the going gets really sucky. Ultimately, support from others can protect you from the three common pitfalls of change: feeling alone, fear, and lack of accountability.

Feeling isolated: Who wants to sleep in a tent alone? Often, when we set a new goal, the enormity of the task can feel overwhelming. We might start to lose motivation, judge ourselves, or give up hope. Hearing how others have conquered the same challenges reassures us that change is possible if we just stay in the game.

Fear: It's scary climbing alone. We need reassurance from our team that it's possible to reach the summit. We may be afraid of failure, or we might think success is out of reach. Those old soundtrack loops can play over and over in our heads, reminding us we aren't good enough or don't have what it takes. Our friends reassure us that we are not alone in our fear. Compassion and positive feedback from family members helps soften our insecurities and improve our confidence.

Lack of accountability: Successful changers tell others what their goals are, and they don't conceal their setbacks. They establish accountability with others and give others permission to challenge them when necessary.

THE RIGHT SUPPORT: ASSEMBLE YOUR TEAM
Unfortunately, sometimes not all your friends are on your side. Some are actually accomplices—sort of like the devil on your shoulder—without really trying to sabotage. Given the opportunity, they might just push you off the mountain, rather than throw you a rope. They see change and are frightened by it, too, or worry that if you change your life, you won't have room for them anymore. There are lots of reasons why some people can't support you when you want or need them to. Learning how to reduce negative influence and capitalize on positive is an important secret to long-term success.

Bad habits and good ones are almost always socially in-fluenced.[2] So, it seems that our friends and family are pretty darn influential in our choices. If you are serious about changing old habits, you might want to consider taking an honest evaluation of the people you hang around with.

Who are the obvious naysayers? These are the people who are outwardly unsupportive of your goals, either be-cause their lifestyle is in opposition to your goal, or because they are competitive with your success.

During your initial phase of change, you might want to consider distancing yourself from the people who don't have your best interest in mind. As you become stronger and more committed to your new habit, you will be less likely to give in to peer pressure.

Some people you know may ride the middle. These are the people who need some convincing—this ball is in your court. Be honest with them about your new goals, and tell them exactly how you need them to support you. You might be surprised by how many people you can influence to be on your team.

Who is on your short list of loyal, unwavering support? These are the people who will stay with you no matter what and will hold you accountable to your goals. Loyalty comes in all shapes and sizes—cheerleaders, nurturers, and the tough coaches. Successful changers know that sometimes we need the tough coach—someone to scream at us, "Why did you do that?" Other times, we need praise or a reassur-ing hug.

STAY ACCOUNTABLE TO YOUR TEAM

Congratulations! You've called forth your dream, created your vision, and set your goals. You're applying mind over

TIP: Keep your team in the loop. Follow these steps:

1. Meet with your supporters in person, and talk with them about your goals—be specific about your support needs.
2. Give everyone on your team a copy of your vision statement, goals, and timelines.
3. Select one person from your team to be your coaching buddy—this is the person to call when you need an extra dose of support and feedback.
4. Send your team updates about your successes and failures—keep them in the loop.
5. Make friends with your mistakes. Your slip-ups truly are the best learning opportunities. Be honest about your setbacks by acknowledging them to yourself and sharing them with others.
6. Solicit feedback from your team. Where can you improve? Where are you already a success?
7. Join a group that supports your new goal. Local gyms, running clubs, and community support groups are great options.
8. Take advantage of technology. Online support programs are available for 24/7 support.

matter and using physical movement to keep your pesky brain from getting stuck. When the climb gets rocky and challenging, your buddy system is in place. Skill power is the name of the game for you. By learning to say no to momentary urges and taking your climb one step at a time, you're well on your way to reaching the top of your mountain.

Changing your behavior and thinking is a critical part of the climb, but without proper fitness and nutrition, you won't make it to the summit. So be sure to read on! You'll meet our in-house expert on everything and anything you need to know about getting your body prepared for a grueling climb (Brian is really the "science guy" for fitness and nutrition, and he'll keep you at the top of that mountain and looking at other horizons and summits).

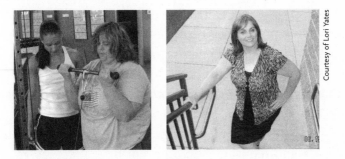

Courtesy of Lori Yates

Get Inspired: Lori Yates's Story

LORI'S MESSAGE: *Diet, exercise, accountability, and a good support system are all that's needed to lose weight, get fit, and stay healthy.*

I had been morbidly obese for many years and struggled with continually gaining weight. I felt horrible about myself. I hated looking in the mirror and seeing my face with three chins. I was depressed. It got so bad that I contemplated suicide. I just felt so overwhelmed. My weight ballooned to 306 pounds, and I was on a diet of fast food and soft drinks. I would eat at home by myself, devouring a large pizza or a dozen cupcakes in one sitting, and then do the same thing the next day and the next.

Then around my forty-fifth birthday, I got the news from my doctor: a diagnosis of diabetes mellitus. This is not happening, I thought. I was scared and angry. I told the doctor that I wasn't going to take medications. He told me I could hold off, if I lost weight and changed my eating habits. I decided I would do it—I would not be diabetic. I knew I had to lose weight and was ready to do something about it. A brand-new Anytime Fitness gym had opened less than a block from the hospital where I work as a clinical social worker. I signed up with a personal trainer who conducted an initial health assessment and developed a nutrition plan for me. Then, I started the workouts. My body hurt, but it didn't hurt nearly as much as my bruised ego. I remembered my younger days, when I could kick out push-ups and sit-ups. Somehow, I was thinking it would be the same, but when I tried to get off the ground, reality hit: I can't get off the floor. Tears rolled down my face. But I told myself, I am not quitting.

Since starting my journey, I have lost one hundred pounds and feel fantastic. I do not have diabetes, my depression and anxiety are well under control, and I am living and enjoying life. I now work out six days a week, and at least four of those days are two-a-day workouts. I do Cross-Fit training twice a week. I ran my first 3½ miles nonstop. I compete against my trainer doing one hundred sit-ups for time, and I can hold my own against her!

I have taken 100 percent responsibility for eating healthy and exercising. I am thankful that I have gone through this experience. I never, ever thought there would be a day that I would love myself, love my body, and love where I am in my life. Now I do.

"Feeling a little pain from a workout is nothing in comparison to feeling shame from being morbidly obese. Take control of your life now, and instead of filling your plate with food, serve yourself energy, esteem, and happiness." —Chuck Runyon

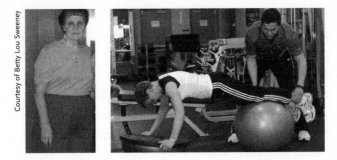

LEFT: Betty Lou. RIGHT: Betty Lou with her trainer, Dave, at the gym.
Courtesy of Anytime Fitness.

Get Inspired: Betty Lou Sweeney's Story

BETTY'S MESSAGE: *Never underestimate yourself because you are all winners, every one of you!*

In 2009, I almost died after a bladder infection reached my heart and threatened to shut down my kidneys. It didn't help that I was 235 pounds at the time or that the infection caused me to gain an additional 35 pounds of water weight. Luckily, I survived and made a promise to myself that if I ever walked out of that hospital, I would make a new start— and commit to getting healthy once and for all.

After noticing an Anytime Fitness near my house, I decided to give a gym membership a try. I started to go to the club three or four times a week, just walking on the treadmill. Eventually, I began working with a personal trainer. And, boy did I luck out with the most amazing trainer, Dave Candra. Dave is twenty-four and I'm seventy-one—but we turned out to be a match made in fitness heaven.

I started training three times a week, barely able to sustain Level 2 on a treadmill. It was incredibly hard, but as the months rolled on, my weight started to drop. Today, after just one year, I have lost 110 pounds and wear a size 4. My life has changed in so many ways. I used to be on twenty-six medications, and now I'm on just three. I wore a swimsuit for the first time in sixty years and sashayed my way onto the national stage with an invitation from the *Today* show! My flexibility and posture have improved, and my joints don't ache anymore.

With such a renewed energy and love for life, I continue to push myself to new heights every day. In fact, I discovered that I have a unique talent for abdominal planking and just recently I shattered the world record* of thirty-three minutes and forty seconds by holding the position for nearly thirty-seven minutes! Not only am I a survivor, but I'm a world champion.

"Remember, a treadmill doesn't care about your age, shape or size. It's ready when you are and if a seventy-one-year-old grandmother can lose 110 pounds and break a world record, I think you can get off your ass!"
—Chuck Runyon

---

*Verification from the *Guinness Book of World Records* pending.

PART 3

NUTRITION SUCKS, TOO, BUT . . .

BRIAN ZEHETNER

So you know that changing your behavior sucks (the *process*, that is—not the changes themselves), but then again, a lot of things suck. You could easily think of something more fun to do when you're flossing your teeth, but you still do it. Why? Because Mom said you should, your dentist will yell at you if you don't, your spouse or partner will make fun of you when offered a spinach-infused smile, and for several other less important reasons. You have to look at eating well in much the same light. Doing what you know you should do nutritionally sort of sucks. After all, it's easy to eat like crap. There aren't really any immediate repercussions for doing so, and the food usually tastes pretty damn good. But then again, we all know the benefits of eating a healthy diet. Knowing this, do we really want poor nutritional habits to be the norm? Probably not.

The real question is, where do we go from here? Nutrition is a science, but we won't delve into the entire body of knowledge on these pages. Instead, we'll focus on a few nutritional topics that are fundamental to both wellness and weight management. Let's get started!

THE CARB CRAZINESS

No other nutrient on the planet has caused more debate among researchers and consumers alike than carbohydrates. Everyone has an opinion when it comes to sugar, high-fructose corn syrup, artificial sweeteners, and various other carb-related topics. To this day, if I happen to mention that I'm a dietitian, I get asked question after question, and most of them are related to carbohydrates. Part of this fervor stems from the resurgence of low-carb diets in the 1990s, which inadvertently set up a war between low-carb addicts and people who saw carbs as part of a healthy diet. But here's the funny thing—the interest and controversy have not gone away. Updated versions of some of the low-carb diet books are coming out, we still have the nutritional establishment touting carbohydrates as an important dietary staple, and then we have consumers stuck in the middle trying to decipher the mixed messages.

Let's cut through the crap. Here's what we know: Carbs are an important energy source, they encompass everything from fruits and vegetables to grains and sugary sweets, they provide four calories per gram, and if you eat too much (of anything, really), you'll probably increase those pesky body fat stores. But do you really know the best sources, how much you should eat, whether you should be concerned about your sugar intake, and whether all those sugar substitutes are dangerous? The next few pages will help you get some answers to these questions.

CARBOHYDRATES ARE HEALTHY, RIGHT?

As you might have guessed, I'm in the camp that believes that carbohydrates are an important part of a healthy diet. And this is especially true if we're talking about fruits, vegetables, beans, and whole grains. Last time I checked, these sources were full of the good stuff, providing plenty of vitamins, minerals, phytonutrients (special plant chemicals that fight disease), and fiber. In other words, these foods pack a serious nutritional punch. And let's not forget that they've

---

Q: What's the difference between whole grains and refined grains?

A: The main difference is the way in which they're processed. During milling, whole grains are often stripped of their bran and germ (two parts of the grain) in an effort to make them easier to cook with. The bran and the germ contribute a number of healthful nutrients, including B vitamins, antioxidants, fiber, healthy fats, and protein. When they're removed, the endosperm is all that is left, which is primarily starch. Despite being enriched with some vitamins and minerals, these refined grains lack much of their original nutritional value. Nowadays, more and more companies are pulverizing the entire grain, resulting in what we call whole-grain products. These are healthier for you, but you have to be a savvy shopper. Look for whole grains listed on the packaging of your favorite products.

been linked to a reduced risk of heart disease, stroke, hypertension, and even some cancers. Armed with this information, you should feel absolutely no need to severely restrict or eliminate these foods from your diet.

SUGAR AIN'T SO SWEET

One thing we have to realize is that sugar is a carbohydrate too, and we take in far too much! But it's not natural sugar, like the kind you find in fruit, that I'm necessarily concerned with. The problem stems from all the added sugars pumped into crackers, doughnuts, cereals, chips, cookies, soda, and almost every other processed food or beverage. Even dried fruit, which is essentially all sugar, often has *added* sugar as well. Don't get me wrong—added sugars aren't much of a concern if consumed in moderation, but therein lies the problem. According to a recent study in the *American Journal of Clinical Nutrition,* average added sugar intake in the United States is about 77 grams per day, or 308 calories. In fact, added sugars make up about 15 percent of total calories in the average diet.[1] Compare this with the American Heart Association recommendation of no more than 100 calories a day from added sugars for women and no more than 150 calories a day for men, and you can see we've clearly got a problem on our hands.[2]

Added sugars have actually been linked to obesity, diabetes, and heart disease, so they're a far cry from the healthy carbohydrates we discussed earlier. Sugar, in all its forms, is really just a source of empty calories, and often displaces much healthier food choices. Therefore, we need to read food labels, watch out for hidden sources, and make every effort to curb our love of the sweet stuff.

But what does this mean in a practical sense? Is it possible to eat some cake, a doughnut, or some cookies and still be healthy? Of course. And life just isn't as fun if you can't have one of your favorite foods every now and then. But somehow, desserts and treats went from a monthly or weekly occurrence decades ago to a daily occurrence today. This type of consumption can easily sabotage your best efforts to stay trim and fit. Rather than stocking your entire pantry with sugary goodies, try purchasing one treat at the store each week, and then indulge once or twice a week. And if sugar creeps into all of your meals and snacks, gradually work on minimizing your intake over a period of several weeks. Here are a few ideas to get you started:

- Buy sugar-free or low-calorie beverages.
- Add fresh or dried fruit to oatmeal, cereals, and yogurt.
- Cut the sugar in your favorite recipes by one-third.
- Add spices and extracts like cinnamon, nutmeg, and vanilla to your dishes instead of sugar.
- Substitute fruit and low-calorie Cool Whip for more traditional sugar-filled desserts.

THE AMOUNT MAKES ALL THE DIFFERENCE

In my fifteen years of working with clients, I've come to an interesting conclusion regarding carbohydrates. Either people seem to overeat carbs to a great degree, or they seem to avoid them like the plague, but very few seem to fall in the middle. This leads us to our next question: How much is necessary for optimal health and wellness? The acceptable macronutrient distribution range (AMDR) is set at 45 to 65 percent of total calories, which means that your carb intake should ideally fall within this range, though there may be exceptions to this rule. So, for example, if you are a woman aiming to eat about 1,500 calories per day, then carbohydrates should make up about 675 to 975 calories (169 to 244 grams of carbohydrate) in your diet. The preceding range is fairly broad and should meet the needs of almost all individuals. Keep in mind, if weight loss is your goal, it's probably a good idea to stay on the lower end. But if you're accustomed to high levels of physical activity, then the higher end may be more appropriate. Ultimately, carbohydrate intake should be tailored to your activity level. The

CHECK THIS OUT!

High-fructose corn syrup (HFCS) has been one of the most controversial nutritional topics in recent years. This engineered carbohydrate is found in everything from bread and soda to jelly and ketchup, and many people are concerned about its safety profile and the implications it may have for long-term health. Let's be clear here—HFCS is not good for you. But if you've been convinced that it poses additional health risks compared with sugar or is simply worse for you from a health perspective, then you may need to rethink things. The scientific evidence indicates that HFCS and sugar affect the body in very similar ways, and there's no reason to limit HFCS any more than other caloric sweeteners.[3] Unfortunately, some health professionals have ignored this research when discussing this issue with the public and the media. Bottom line—avoid HFCS because it's considered a source of empty calories, but not because it poses more health risks than traditional sugar.

more active you are, the more carbohydrates you can and should eat. Check out the following tips for incorporating quality carbs into your eating plan.

- Consume some sort of grain (ideally a whole grain) at each meal, and experiment with different options.
- Include at least one serving of fruit at breakfast, lunch, and dinner (or as a dessert after dinner).
- Add one glass of 100 percent juice for breakfast, but avoid other sugar-containing beverages when possible.
- Aim for one serving of two different vegetables at both lunch and dinner.
- Try to incorporate beans in at least two to three meals each week. There are plenty of good choices, including navy beans, kidney beans, black beans, and pinto beans.
- Limit your intake of cookies, chips, and other processed snack foods. Go for fruits, vegetables, whole-grain crackers, or plain yogurt instead.

SWEET CONTROVERSY

Two issues that are fairly controversial and receive a lot of attention involve the use of artificial sweeteners and sugar alcohols as replacements for good ol' sugar. If you choose a food product off the store shelf, there's a good chance that it contains one of these sugar replacements. They're everywhere, and the medical establishment is partly to blame. Doctors have done a pretty good job of scaring us away from sugar in all its forms. Some medical professionals agree with these scare tactics and are very concerned about excessive sugar consumption, while others argue that these sugar substitutes actually pose a greater risk to health. So what does the research say?

On average, artificial sweeteners and sugar alcohols have proven to be safe for most people. In fact, people with diabetes regularly use these substitutes so they can indulge in the occasional sweet without affecting their blood sugar levels. Some folks do experience adverse reactions to certain sweeteners, but this is the exception and not the rule. You've probably noticed that companies are moving toward new age sweeteners like sucralose (Splenda) and stevia (Truvia). There are still plenty of products that use the more traditional artificial sweeteners as well, but these two seem to be winning the popularity contest. I'm fine with either one and have no problem recommending them to my clients. But the bottom line is, you have a choice. You can eat products with artificial sweeteners, or you can avoid them altogether. Whatever you decide, just make sure your decision is based on sound science.

GO FIBER
OR GO HOME

Fiber is essentially nature's version of human Drano. It helps to clean out your internal system (your gastrointestinal tract), and for years, we really didn't think it played any other significant role in health. Were we ever wrong! Fiber is now known to have several health benefits, many of which we'll discuss. But first, let's figure out what it is, how much you need, and where you can find it.

HOW DO YOU TAKE YOURS?
Fiber is a mix of complex carbohydrates that the body can't digest and absorb, at least not to any great degree. So for our purposes, it's basically a calorie-free bulking agent. These long chains of carbohydrate pass through the gastrointestinal (GI) tract without being converted into energy, and it is this characteristic of fiber that's key to the health benefits it provides.

Fiber is a really a general term that encompasses two primary categories. Soluble fiber dissolves in water to become a viscous, gummy mess, and this mess is what contributes to fiber's health-promoting properties. On the other hand, insoluble fiber actually holds on to water and moves waste through the GI tract quicker.

FINDING THE RIGHT BALANCE

Americans eat around 12 to 18 grams of fiber today, which is far below the levels recommended by the Food and Nutrition Board of the National Academy of Sciences.[1] The dietary reference intake for men aged nineteen to fifty is 38 grams per day, and for women of the same age, it's 25 grams per day.[2] In other words, our collective fiber intake is awful and is most likely attributed to our poor intake of fruits and vegetables, among other things. We're too busy sucking down burgers, fries, pizza, and chicken wings to worry about the healthy stuff. As a matter of fact, we don't eat enough whole grains, nuts, seeds, and beans, let alone the aforementioned fruits and vegetables, which all happen to be excellent sources of fiber.

So does this mean that we should all be consuming fiber supplements as though they're going out of style? Not so fast. If we make some simple dietary changes and eat what we all know we probably should eat on a daily basis, fiber supplements aren't needed. Don't get me wrong; supplements do have their place for people who have aversions to some of the best fiber sources or for people experiencing GI problems, but for most of us, real food works just fine.

Though most folks fall on the low end of the totem pole, it is possible to take in *too much* fiber as well. If you do take in too much—on the order of 50 or 60 grams per day or more—you may experience increased gas, bloating, and diarrhea, not to mention reduced absorption of several key vitamins and minerals. So for the great majority of us, we should try to improve our intake, but we need to be careful about overdoing it.

CHECK THIS OUT!

Here's a list of some everyday foods that contain fiber.* Remember, most of us fall short of our daily goal, but if you add some of these to your other dietary staples, you'll hit the recommendation in no time!

Food	*Fiber (in grams)*
½ cup navy beans	9.6
½ cup kidney beans	6.5
1 ounce bran flakes	5.3
Medium pear	5.1
½ cup peas	4.4
½ cup raspberries	4.0
Medium baked potato (with skin)	3.8
¼ cup sunflower seeds	3.6
3 cups popcorn	3.5
Medium apple	3.3
Medium banana	3.1
½ cup broccoli	2.6
½ cup oatmeal (cooked)	2.0
¼ cup walnuts	2.0
1 slice whole wheat bread	1.9
1 medium carrot	1.7
½ cup brown rice (cooked)	1.8

*From U.S. Department of Agriculture, Agricultural Research Service, USDA Nutrient Data Laboratory, "USDA National Nutrient Database for Standard Reference," Release 23, 2010.

THE UNSUNG HERO OF HEALTH

Insoluble fiber is known to make the stool soft and bulky (a lovely thought), which promotes regularity and prevents constipation. This speedy transit also happens to reduce the contact time that toxins and chemicals may have with the GI tract—an added bonus. Soluble fiber, on the other hand, actually helps to lower your cholesterol level. People who take in a lot of fiber seem to have a lower risk of cancer as well. Fiber may even be advantageous to those with diabetes. But one of the most interesting aspects of fiber is its effect on weight management. Fiber-rich foods are ideal for weight-conscious consumers for three reasons:

- They are often lower in calories, fat, and added sugars.
- They take longer to chew, which means you'll be likely to eat slower.
- They are bulky, which could contribute to an earlier feeling of fullness (this has to do with a concept called energy density, which we'll cover more extensively in the weight management chapter).

All of this adds up to eating less food and consuming fewer calories, which, as we all know, is pretty damn important for weight loss.

There are several health claims that can be made for foods containing fiber. Keep in mind that health claims typically require significant scientific agreement, so the basis for these claims is pretty strong.[3] Check out the following list.

- Low-fat diets rich in fiber-containing grain products, fruits, and vegetables may reduce the risk of some types of cancer.
- Diets low in saturated fat and cholesterol and rich in fruits, vegetables, and grain products that contain some types of dietary fiber, particularly soluble fiber, may reduce the risk of heart disease.
- Soluble fiber, as part of a diet low in saturated fat and cholesterol, may reduce the risk of heart disease.

And these aren't the only claims that can be made about fiber. There's also an easy way to identify those foods that are considered decent sources. A food that's considered high in fiber has 5 or more grams per serving, and a food labeled a "good source of fiber" has 2.5 to 4.9 grams per serving.

PROTEIN: THE PERFECT BUILDING MATERIAL

You've probably been to a local gym sometime and over-heard the heavily muscled dudes talking about protein. It's a conversation that occurs almost every day. And if you've been privy to one of these conversational nuggets, you've probably heard one of the guys rattle off his protein intake for the day. It usually goes something like this: twelve egg whites for breakfast, two 8-ounce chicken breasts for lunch, two cups of cottage cheese for his afternoon snack, and a 10-ounce flank steak for dinner. Oh, and did I forget the two protein shakes as well? Just FYI, this is close to 400 grams of protein per day, and accounts for almost 1,600 calories from this one nutrient! How's that for balance and modera-tion, huh?

Protein is definitely an important factor in the muscle-building process, but it also serves several other important functions in the body. Most of these relate to the mainte-nance and repair of tissues. It also provides four calories per gram, just like carbohydrates, and can be used for en-ergy in certain circumstances. With these basic facts out of the way, let's turn our attention to more important matters. How much do you actually need on a daily basis, and where can you get it? And let's bust a few myths along the way too.

TOO MUCH, TOO LITTLE, OR JUST RIGHT?

Interestingly, if you search for protein recommendations on the Internet, you'll come across a ton of results advocating 2 grams per pound (yes, per *pound*) for weight lifters and other active individuals. This is simply ridiculous. There's absolutely no need to take in that much protein daily. Despite this reality, plenty of people still follow this recommendation. What they don't realize is that after the body's protein needs are met, the excess will either be used as an energy source or be stored as fat. And then there's the concern that kidney and liver function will deteriorate when protein intake gets to this level. Luckily, there isn't any research indicating that high-protein diets hurt people who are healthy, but there's an important caveat here that we shouldn't ignore. How do you know if you have normal kidney and liver function? Do you really know if your kidneys and liver are working as well as they should be? Many folks in the early stages of disease are asymptomatic and

---

CHECK THIS OUT!

One of the biggest myths in sports nutrition is the idea that an individual can digest only 30 grams of protein per meal. Some think Lou Ferrigno (of *The Incredible Hulk* fame) came up with this little ditty while training in Gold's Gym back in the day, but no one knows for sure. Regardless, this statement is completely false. You can digest and absorb as much protein as you can eat in one sitting. However, the key point here is that the more you eat, the longer the digestive process is going to take.

completely unaware of the potential for problems down the road. In the end, we need to be more rational when it comes to our own protein intake and ignore the Internet chatter.

Thankfully, a few guidelines can help us determine our protein needs. First of all, the acceptable macronutrient distribution range (AMDR) for protein is 10 to 35 percent of daily calories. But because of the increasing popularity of sports nutrition over the past few decades, scientists started studying the protein needs for individuals engaging in varying levels of physical activity, with the goal of offering more specific recommendations. The guidelines established as a result of this research are still used to this day and provide a nice guide for those of us who may not have a clue as to how much protein we should eat. Check out the chart below to see where you fit in.

Level of Activity	Daily Protein Intake (grams per pound of body weight)
Sedentary	0.36
Active adults (recreational exercisers)	0.36–0.45
Endurance athletes	0.54–0.63
Strength athletes	0.73–0.77
Strength athletes (during weight loss)	0.91

Basically, if you aren't all that active, you probably need the recommended dietary allowance of 0.36 grams of protein per pound of body weight (e.g., that's about 8 ounces of meat or the equivalent per day for a 154-pound person). Those who are training for cardiovascular endurance need a bit more, simply because of the increased demands on the body, and if you're looking to add significant muscle mass

DID YOU KNOW?

Theoretically, it takes only an *additional* 14 grams of protein per day to build 1 pound of muscle per week. That's right, only 14 grams! Here's how the math breaks down:

1 pound = 454 grams
Muscle is approximately 22 percent protein, so
    454 × 0.22 = 100 grams of protein in 1 pound of muscle
Dividing 100 grams by 7 days per week = 14 grams of
    protein per day

You can easily consume this amount of protein in a glass of milk and 1 ounce of meat, so again, there's no need to go overboard on protein, even if building muscle is your primary goal.

Check out the protein content of some of your favorite foods:[1]

Food	Grams of Protein
3 oz. flank steak	30
3 oz. chicken	26
3 oz. tuna	23
3 oz. salmon	20
¼ cup peanuts	10
½ cup beans	8
8 oz. milk	8
1 oz. cheddar cheese	7
8 oz. low-fat yogurt	6
1 baked potato	5
1 slice whole wheat bread	3
½ cup brown rice	2.5
½ cup spinach	2.5
½ cup broccoli	2

and size, then you probably need even more. Interestingly, people looking to lose weight are often advised to increase their protein intake slightly. The reason for this is because it can be difficult to maintain muscle tissue in the face of a caloric deficit. Losing muscle is not ideal, so if you're looking to drop a few pounds, increasing your protein a bit may help to prevent this scenario as the weight comes off. In other words, if you're a recreational exerciser taking in approximately 0.45 grams of protein per pound, but you're actively losing weight, it might be advisable to increase your protein intake to 0.54 grams per pound, which amounts to an additional 2 ounces of meat or the equivalent per day. This same principle applies to all individuals, regardless of activity level.

WHERE ART THOU, PROTEIN?
It's a simple fact—protein is available in a wide variety of foods. Meats, poultry, and seafood are all excellent sources, along with eggs and dairy products. But you can't forget about vegetarian sources as well, which can contribute significantly to overall protein intake. Beans, nuts and seeds, and legumes are all good sources, and even grain products and vegetables add protein to the diet. And then you have all the protein powders and engineered sports nutrition products, too (check out the supplement chapter "To Supplement or Not, That Is the Question" for more information). Most of us should have no problem meeting our daily protein needs, given all of these options. And as long as you try to follow the principles of balance, variety, and moderation, you'll be likely to do it in the healthiest way possible.

SIMPLIFYING THE FATS ISN'T SO SIMPLE

It's always the good stuff: From chicken wings to french fries and ice cream to the latest fried state fair treats, we're literally surrounded by good-tasting, high-fat food. And we wonder why overweight and obesity are at such epic proportions. After all, fat does have 9 calories per gram, which is over twice that of carbohydrate and protein. This means that high-fat foods typically have more calories, and as a result, high-fat diets have traditionally been pretty good at packing on the pounds. But interestingly, our attitudes toward dietary fat have changed dramatically over the years.

Dietary fat has quite the interesting story to tell. Decades ago, people really paid little attention to the fat content of their diets. People ate what they wanted to, and that was it—end of story. Then, they starting hearing warnings about fat intake, cholesterol levels, and cardiovascular disease, and people took notice. Companies began slashing the fat content of their foods, and low and behold, the low-fat era was born. Gradually, more and more research was conducted, and scientists soon discovered that certain fats were actually beneficial to health. Recommendations changed, and health professionals starting educating people about the potential benefits of substances like omega-3 fatty acids, polyunsaturated fats, and monounsaturated fats, while also highlighting the dangers of saturated and trans fats. This same philosophical approach is used by doctors and dietitians to this day, but there are still some health professionals on the fringe that don't see a need for limits on *any* of these fats. And so the story continues . . .

As you can see, nothing in nutrition is simple, and that's certainly true of dietary fats. It's a pretty complicated topic, so let's stick to two important issues: the optimal amount of fat to consume in the diet and a brief discussion about the types of fats and how they affect your health.

QUANTITY VERSUS QUALITY

The amount of fat in the diet can vary greatly among individuals. Some people are convinced that high intakes of dietary fat equate to high levels of body fat (which isn't necessarily true), so they limit fat intake as much as possible. Others buy into the fast-food lifestyle or simply don't pay attention to the fat content of the foods they eat, so they end up with relatively high intakes in comparison. The acceptable macronutrient distribution range (AMDR) for fat is 20 to 35 percent of total calories. This guideline is certainly reasonable, but surprisingly, more people seem to be concerned about the levels of carbohydrate and protein in their diets. So rather than diligently trying to figure out exactly how much fat they should take in, most people simply figure out their carbohydrate and protein needs, and then let fat make up the remainder of the calories. Luckily, for most people, their fat intake will still fall within the AMDR. It's important to try to avoid high-fat diets in general, especially those that are high in unhealthy fats, since these fats have been linked

DID YOU KNOW?

Low-fat doesn't necessarily mean low-calorie. Foods that have a lower fat content would certainly seem to be lower in calories, given the fact that fats provide 9 calories per gram, versus 4 calories per gram for both carbohydrates and proteins. However, in many of the low-fat products on the market, manufacturers simply add additional carbohydrates to replace some of the missing flavor and texture that fats provide. In many cases, this leaves the food with about the same number of calories as the original version, and sometimes even more. The bottom line is, you need to be a savvy label reader. Try to compare regular versions of your favorite products with their low-fat counterparts to see if they're truly a healthy alternative.

to obesity, cardiovascular disease, and even certain cancers. Now let's consider some very important topics—the types of fats, where you can find them, and their effects on health. It's important to note that most of our food examples in the following section contain several types of fats, but one type usually predominates.

SATURATED FATS

These types of fats primarily come from animal-based foods such as meats, poultry, butter, whole milk, and even from coconut and palm oils. They're also found in a wide variety of processed food products, and thankfully, the saturated fat content of these foods is known because these fats are listed on the nutrition facts panel on food labels. Saturated fats are usually solid at room temperature and are known to increase both total cholesterol and "bad" LDL (low-density lipoprotein) cholesterol. Because of this, these fats are linked to an increased risk for heart attack and stroke. Therefore, the general recommendation is to consume less than 10 percent of total calories as saturated fats. Note that saturated fats (and trans fats as well) actually affect blood cholesterol levels more than does the cholesterol we consume from foods.

You may be wondering why LDL cholesterol is considered bad and HDL (high-density lipoprotein) cholesterol is considered good. Here's the scoop: LDL's job is to take cholesterol and other fats to the body's cells. En route, LDL particles can get stuck in your arteries and form plaques that block blood flow, a condition that could ultimately lead to a heart attack or stroke. Higher levels of LDL are associated with a higher risk for both of these events. HDL, on the other hand, is beneficial because it carries cholesterol and other fats from the body's cells back to the liver for processing and excretion. Therefore, high HDL levels are associated with a reduced risk for heart attack and stroke. HDL levels can be difficult to increase, but aerobic exercise, mild alcohol consumption, and increased monounsaturated fat intake may help, along with quitting smoking and losing weight.

TRANS FATS

Trans fats can be found in foods naturally, but you'll often see them in heavily processed foods as a result of a complicated process called hydrogenation. This process makes fats firmer, which helps to extend the shelf life of many prepackaged items. Unfortunately, trans fats have an effect similar to that of saturated fats, increasing total and LDL cholesterol and possibly decreasing "good" HDL cholesterol. The same risks for heart attack and stroke apply as well. Your best bet is to avoid trans fats entirely. Look to avoid products that contain partially hydrogenated vegetable oil, which indicates the presence of trans fats. You can also find trans fats listed on the nutrition facts panel on food labels.

POLYUNSATURATED FATS
Polyunsaturated fats are usually liquid at room temperature and encompass most of the vegetable oils that you're probably familiar with. These include corn, safflower, soybean, sesame, and sunflower oils. Seafood is actually a very good source as well. These particular fats fall in the middle when it comes to heart health. They decrease total and LDL cholesterol, which is great, but they also have the potential to decrease HDL.

MONOUNSATURATED FATS
You can find this these types of fats in canola oil, olive oil, and several nut oils, including peanut oil. Monounsaturated fats are responsible for decreasing total and LDL cholesterol, and they may even increase HDL. Therefore, this type of fat is clearly a winner when it comes to heart health.

OMEGA-3 FATTY ACIDS
The two primary omega-3 fatty acids are EPA and DHA, which are found in fatty fish like salmon, mackerel, and tuna. There's also a third fatty acid, ALA, which can be converted to EPA and DHA to a small degree. ALA is found in walnuts and in soy, canola, and flaxseed oils. Omega-3 fatty acids actually decrease triglycerides (the fats in our blood)

and may decrease total cholesterol as well. They have also been shown to prevent blood from clotting and sticking to artery walls. For more information on the benefits of omega-3 fatty acids, check out the supplement chapter "To Supplement or Not, That Is the Question."

Sadly, the typical American diet does not lend itself to heart health and the prevention of cardiovascular disease. The most prevalent fats in our food supply are not necessarily the healthiest types. Therefore, it might be wise to change up the types of oils you use in your cooking, consume a bit more fatty fish, increase your intake of nuts and seeds (and other vegetarian food options like soy), and significantly decrease your intake of processed foods. If you can incorporate some of these relatively basic changes into your diet, you'll be better off in the long run. For additional tips on substituting healthier fats, check out the practical recommendations found at the beginning of the last chapter in this book, "Your 21-Day Nutrition and Fitness Plan."

THE OMEGA-6:OMEGA-3 RATIO

Another very important issue that garners little attention involves the ratio of omega-6 to omega-3 fatty acids in our diets and how this affects immune function and overall health. In the Paleolithic era (think hunter-gatherers), the omega-6:omega-3 ratio of humans was about 1:1, meaning people ate about as much of the omega-3 fatty acids as they did the omega-6 ones. But can you guess what that ratio is today in the typical American diet? Approximately 15:1![1] That's right, we now eat 15 times as much omega-6 fatty acids. So the real question is, what effect does this have on our long-term health?

Polyunsaturated fats (which include omega-3 and omega-6 fatty acids) are known to affect immune function, that is, how the body reacts to perceived foreign entities like germs or foreign tissue. In short, omega-6, most typically found in vegetable oils like corn, soybean, and safflower, is generally considered to be pro-inflammatory. And in the short term (think a minor injury), inflammation is a good thing. But—and this is a big but (no pun intended)—it can wreak havoc on the body if it continues chronically. Omega-3 fatty acids, on the other hand, are considered anti-inflammatory. So essentially, this means we're living in a pro-inflammatory environment, which is not ideal for long-term health. In fact, many scientists and doctors are convinced that heart disease, diabetes, Alzheimer's, cancer, and many other chronic diseases are inflammatory disorders and that lowering the omega-6:omega-3 ratio will reduce the prevalence of these disorders.

It's clear what we have to do. Ideally, we would increase our intake of omega-3's and cut down on our intake of omega-6's, but in the fast-food environment we live in, this is easier said than done. There just aren't that many great sources of omega-3 fatty acids in the food supply. That's why omega-3 supplements like fish oil and flaxseed oil have become so popular. At the very least, we need to stop consuming so many processed foods, because the great majority of them contain vegetable oils high in omega-6's. If we eat a greater amount of naturally occurring foods, we might be able to lower the omega-6:omega-3 ratio, which would result in better health.

THE 411 ON H$_2$O

Our bodies are roughly 60 percent water (males having about 10 percent more body water than females), though you wouldn't know it looking at us. Water serves several important functions in the body, including transporting nutrients and waste, regulating body temperature, and cushioning our joints and organs, among other things. In fact, it's vital to our survival—we can live without food for four to six weeks, but only about one week without some form of water.

PLEASE SHUT UP ABOUT WATER

But I'm not going to lie to you—water sucks. I hate drinking it. It's just too plain, and, shockingly, it tastes like . . . water. But do you know what's even worse? The number of people telling me to drink even more of it. You're tired? Try some water. Hyperactive? Maybe you need some water. Shin splints? Water to the rescue! Despite my distaste for the most abundant natural resource on the planet, it is incredibly important to our overall health and well-being. And you have to get your eight 8-ounce glasses a day, right? Think again. Did you know that there is *no* scientific evidence to support this recommendation? None, nada, zilch. How can this be? There are actually two prevailing theories about how 8 × 8 came to be. The first involves some guy's off-handed comment in some textbook written back in 1974 (seriously), and the other involves a slight misinterpretation of a recommendation by the Food and Nutrition Board of the National Research Council back in 1945.[1] Regardless of which one is right, one true question remains: How much water do *you* need to drink on a daily basis?

JUST GIVE ME THE RECOMMENDATION, ALREADY

The latest dietary reference intake report from the Food and Nutrition Board of the Institute of Medicine contains general fluid recommendations for both men and women. Men should be aiming for 3.7 liters per day, or 125 ounces, while women should shoot for 2.7 liters, or 91 ounces per day.[2] That sounds like a lot, but guess what? The panel noted that prolonged physical activity and hot and humid environmental conditions can increase these numbers even further. Keep in mind, these recommendations come from national data and represent total water from both foods and fluids. In

---

CHECK THIS OUT!

We all know that water has numerous benefits, and research has indicated it can even help with weight loss. A recent study evaluated the effect of drinking water before meals in those following a low-calorie diet. The results were fantastic! The water group lost an average of 2 kilograms (4.4 pounds) of body weight more than the non-water group over twelve weeks.[3] Not bad for a little H$_2$O, huh? The water seems to reduce the amount of calories consumed at the following meal, so if you're looking to drop a few pounds, drink a glass or two before you eat.

fact, they even include beverages containing caffeine and alcohol, since the panel concluded that they contribute to overall hydration if they're consumed in moderation.

So how much should *you* consume each day? Thankfully, there's a very simple formula that you can use to determine the amount of fluid (notice I didn't say water) that you should drink each day. The overriding principle here is that you should base fluid needs on your body weight. Therefore, if you drink half your body weight in ounces, you're getting pretty close. This amount approximates the fluid lost from four bodily processes: breathing, sweating, peeing, and pooping. But you're not done yet. You actually only *drink* about 80 percent of the fluids you take in, with the other 20 percent coming from food. So, you should drink 80 percent of that original number.

SO IS IT WATER OR SOMETHING ELSE?

You know that water is important for health, and you know about how much you should drink, but you're probably curious about what to drink. Luckily, this is an easy one. Water is clearly your best option, and I say this as someone who really dislikes plain water, as I mentioned earlier. And water is definitely the answer if you're looking to lose a few pounds, since drinking excess calories is a surefire way to derail your weight loss efforts. But if you're like me, and plain water is one of your last options and calories aren't a huge issue for you, then stick with skim milk, teas, and all-natural fruit juices to satisfy your daily water needs. You get a dose of nutrition with these guys in the form of vitamins, minerals, and antioxidants, so you really can't go wrong. There's a place for sports drinks as well, though this assumes you're

THE 411 ON H$_2$O

DID YOU KNOW?

Like our bodies, many foods are also composed of water. Check out the water content of these popular dietary staples.[4] Some of them might surprise you!

Food	Percentage of Water
Lettuce	95
Milk	89
Apple	86
Potato	75
Kidney beans	67
Beef	64
Whole wheat bread	38
Cheddar cheese	37
Margarine	16
Pecans	4
Vegetable oil	0

engaging in prolonged, intense physical activities that require additional energy. If this isn't the case, then you can probably avoid this category of beverages altogether.

I know what you coffee fans are thinking. When is he going to demonize my morning pick-me-up? Well, Starbucks fans, rejoice! Moderate coffee consumption (maybe a cup or two a day) is fine for most folks and actually contributes to your daily water total as well. But I'm talking about coffee here and not the 600-calorie espresso desserts that you can buy on almost any street corner. Let's use common sense, people. The caramel-infused, whole-milk-coffee combos with real whipped cream on top are not the answer when it comes to hydration, and you know it!

DID YOU KNOW?

The average American consumes 44.7 gallons of soft drinks each year, according to a recent *New York Times* article by Mark Bittman.[5] And this doesn't even include noncarbonated sweetened beverages, which amount to another 17 gallons per person per year! Bittman points out that by 2001, Americans were consuming 278 more daily calories than they were in 1977, and 40 percent of those extra calories came from soda, fruit drinks, sports drinks, and mixes like Kool-Aid. Unfortunately, there are some serious marketing dollars behind all of these products, so it could be awhile before we see these numbers drop significantly.

There are a few beverages that could clearly contribute to your total water intake, but sadly, they're on the limit or avoid list. The aforementioned coffee dessert comes to mind, but I'm also talking about soft drinks (diet and regular), alcohol, and energy drinks (and anything else I've forgotten to mention). Excessive sugar, alcohol, and all those energy drink ingredients that you can't pronounce—these are by no means the pillars of nutrition. I am a realist, however, and I know that an occasional soda or beer isn't going to cause any major problems. But when it comes to hydration, there are simply better options. So if you're relying on any one of these to get you through your day, try switching to water or one of your other favorites.

TO SUPPLEMENT OR NOT, THAT IS THE QUESTION

I might be stating the obvious here, but supplement use has gotten out of control. In fact, the only thing that has gotten more out of control than the supplements is the marketing for the supplements. You've seen the commercials for 5-hour ENERGY, right? Some dreary-eyed fellow drags his butt out of bed complaining about his early alarm and the workday ahead, only to open the cupboard and find the perfect pick-me-up. And after sucking down his little energy shot, he's running down the stairs bright-eyed, bushy-tailed, and ready to take on all comers. Who knew we were in the midst of an energy crisis—one that didn't involve that black, tarry stuff buried underground?

WE'VE GOT AN ADDICTION

Don't get me wrong, though; it's not all about energy in a bottle. We also have a serious infatuation with fat-burners, protein powders, multivitamins, and antioxidant juices, to name just a few. And unfortunately, people buy into the marketing hype, to the tune of $26.9 billion a year.[1] That's what I call *big* business. With that amount of money rolling in, you can only imagine the number of supplement categories and the thousands of individual products in each.

So where does that leave us? It's clear that we should all follow a "food first" philosophy, but supplements can and do play a role in health and wellness. Rather than giving you an encyclopedia of supplement info that'll make your eyes glaze over, let's discuss a few of what I like to call "foundational supplements" that may benefit health or performance. We'll also briefly cover some of the most popular supplements that have little or no impact on health or performance, despite their claims to the contrary. In the end, the goal is to arm yourself with the basic information you need to make an informed decision about your own use of dietary supplements. Are you ready?

THE GOOD GUYS

Despite the obvious problems of relying on overhyped supplements as a substitute for bad nutrition, certain supplements can provide health and performance benefits when they are used intelligently. That's the key—to be knowledgeable about what is going inside your body. Check out our list of safe and potentially beneficial supplements below.

Multivitamins and Minerals

Multivitamin and mineral supplements (MVIs) are by far the most popular dietary supplement, with approximately 40 percent of men and women over age twenty taking an MVI pill daily.[2] Interestingly, taking an MVI has typically been considered a wise decision by most health professionals. Doctors and dietitians recommended them as an insurance policy of sorts—something that helped fill in any nutritional gaps. But the tide seems to be turning a bit. Now, more and more scientists are saying that MVIs are simply not necessary. They point out that a well-balanced, varied

DID YOU KNOW?

Dietary supplements can be marketed without prior testing for efficacy and safety. Sadly, they are not held to the same standards that are applied to food additives and pharmaceutical drugs. And get this: A dietary supplement is taken off the market only *after* it's been proven to be unsafe. The real problem here is that proving a claim brought against a supplement manufacturer rests with the federal government, specifically the FDA. Somehow, the entire burden has been taken off the manufacturers. I don't think this is the best way to protect consumers, but for now, this is how the system works. These issues highlight the importance of educating yourself and making informed decisions when it comes to your use of dietary supplements.

diet provides all of the essential nutrients that a person needs for optimal health.

Although these scientists have a valid point, how many people actually eat a well-balanced, varied diet? Most folks go to the grocery store and buy the same dietary staples week after week and month after month; many of us eat a fairly monotonous diet of our favorite foods, whether they're good for us or not. For this reason, a simple MVI that provides at least 100 percent of the Recommended Dietary Allowance (RDA) is still warranted. After all, there's really no downside to taking one. In most cases, your body will use what it needs, and eliminate what it doesn't. The hard part is finding the right supplement. You should look for an MVI that is broad-spectrum, meaning it has a comprehensive list of essential nutrients that your body needs on a daily basis. You should also look for products that are manufactured by

reputable companies that follow good manufacturing prac-
tices and FDA regulations. There are plenty of well-formu-
lated products on the market. If you need help choosing the
one that's right for you, talk to a registered dietitian.

Omega-3 Fatty Acids

These fatty acids offer a number of health benefits, and if
experts had to choose between recommending omega-3
supplementation or a daily MVI, some professionals would
probably steer you toward the omega-3's. (For a reminder
on the importance of these fatty acids, check out the earlier
chapter on fats.) Omega-3 fatty acids have been shown to
lower triglycerides levels, reduce risks of heart attack and
stroke, slow the buildup of artery plaques, and slightly lower
blood pressure. And as if that weren't enough, these fatty
acids have also been studied extensively for their neuropro-
tective effects related to Parkinson's disease, Alzheimer's
disease, and depression. If you decide to supplement, your
best bet would be to purchase fish oil because it has a high
concentration of both EPA and DHA. If you're a vegetarian,
getting these two fatty acids becomes a bit more challenging, but look for an algae-based omega-3 product or
flaxseed oil as alternatives. Typical dosages start at 1,000
milligrams of EPA and DHA combined per day for general
health and wellness, and then increase further, depending
on your risk factors for chronic disease.

Sports Drinks

You might find it odd that sports drinks (think Gatorade)
are included in the supplement section, but if you think
about it logically, they belong here. After all, they're designed to help improve performance and they actually work

quite well. But when is it beneficial to use a sports drink, as opposed to plain water or some other beverage? The average person who works out for sixty minutes or less will need nothing more than water to get through a workout. Your body has all the fuel it needs to exercise for that long, especially if you start the workout well fueled—and you should! It really comes down to your goals and the type of workout you're doing to reach those goals. If optimal performance is your focus, or if the planned workout is very intense or more than an hour, then sports drinks are a wise choice. In these instances, your body will need the extra sugar calories—a principal energy source—and electrolytes. In fact, research has proven this over and over again. Most sports drinks are a 6 to 10 percent carbohydrate solution with added sodium and potassium, but formulas do vary. These drinks are specifically designed to be digested and absorbed quickly, so there's no need to dilute them, though this is a common practice amongst novice exercisers and athletes. And don't be too concerned about using a particular product. They all contain water, some form of sugar, and some electrolytes, so find the one you like, and stick with it.

Sports Nutrition Bars

Sports nutrition bars are very popular, and for good reason. They're convenient, generally affordable, and a quick source of on-the-go energy. Depending on the circumstance, they actually work well as either a preworkout snack or a postworkout recovery food. The only real problem is that there are so many options out there, and not all bars are created equal, from a nutritional standpoint. You really need to fine-tune what you're looking for. If you're using these bars before or after your workout, then you should probably look for one that has around 200 to 300 calories, 25 to 35 grams of carbohydrate, 15 to 25 grams of protein, and 3 to 8 grams of fat. Keep in mind, these are just ballpark numbers; the bar you choose could have more or less, depending on your personal preference. A bar that meets these specifications could be used sixty to ninety minutes before your workout or immediately after as a recovery option. Another thing you really need to consider when choosing a bar—and it's a big one—is the taste. Start with the most popular bars first, and then work your way through the myriad of options until you find your personal favorite.

Protein Powders

You can find protein powders everywhere these days, from GNC stores and Internet wholesalers to Walmart and Target—and a lot of people purchase them. But is the additional protein actually needed? The answer to this question really depends on your current eating habits. Most people eat plenty of protein to maintain and repair their bodies on a daily basis, and they probably eat more than enough to stimulate new muscle growth as well, assuming they're training with that goal in mind. However, there's no denying the convenience factor that protein powders afford, and they can help to balance out meals that are traditionally high in carbohydrate and low in protein—specifically, breakfast. Even I've been known to put a little protein powder in my oatmeal every now and then. It's also easy to toss some protein powder into a homemade smoothie right after you finish your workout. Doing this may help you recover from your workout a little faster, which is always a good thing. Ultimately, protein powders are a nice-to-have, but aren't necessarily a need-to-have, so the decision is up to you. If you're looking for a protein powder, try to find a pure form with very few additives. The ideal product should have 15 to 25 grams per serving, with very little carbohydrate or fat. Common sources include whey, casein, egg, soy, and rice.

Creatine

Creatine is one of the pillars of the sports supplement industry. It continues to be incredibly popular among strength training enthusiasts and is still considered a safe and effective supplement for those looking to improve speed, strength, and power. There are literally hundreds of clinical trials on creatine. More recently, researchers have even turned their attention to chronic conditions such as congestive heart failure and several of the neuromuscular diseases. You can still find creatine monohydrate (or some variation) on store shelves, but the trend these days is to include it in a more comprehensive formula with a number of other ingredients that may or may not have creatine's safety and efficacy profile. Regardless, if your goal is to dramatically increase strength and size, I would certainly recommend giving it a try, if you haven't already. However, you need to decide whether to use it on its own or to try one of the complex formulas that contain creatine. If it's the latter, make sure you do your homework on the specific product you choose. Remember, you can always ask a sports dietitian about the proper dosing and timing of creatine and whether you need to cycle on and off over time.

Caffeine

Are you surprised to find caffeine on the good list? Ironically enough, if you're looking for a little pick-me-up before your morning workout, and for whatever reason, you don't like to eat before exercising, then coffee (caffeine) is an excellent alternative. Caffeine is considered a central nervous system stimulant and will provide a boost of energy, though the effect varies greatly among individuals. It's actually considered an ergogenic aid, meaning it enhances physical performance. In the right amounts, caffeine has been shown to reduce the perception of effort during a workout, which means your workout will seem easier than it actually is.[3] As a result, you'll typically perform better! Not bad for a little cup o' joe, huh? Keep in mind, coffee does increase heart rate, respiratory rate, and blood pressure, and it can make you a bit jittery if you're a newbie. Luckily, these effects are relatively mild, especially for healthy folks. In fact, much of the research these days is focused on the potential health benefits of coffee and caffeine, rather than any health risks.

THE BAD GUYS

Some supplements are not worth the money or the health risk. At their worst, they can have side effects, and at their best, they may do nothing. A consumer would be wise to think twice before spending money on these supplements.

Fat Burners

Numerous products on the market contain *thermogenic* ingredients, or what most of us call "fat burners." Ephedrine, yohimbine, green tea extract (EGCG), and bitter orange (synephrine) are examples, and they basically work by stimulating the central nervous system. This increases your fight-or-flight responses, indirectly providing energy and allowing you to process calories at a faster rate. Along with these supposed benefits, there are also side effects associ-

CHECK THIS OUT!

You've all seen those crazy before and after pictures for weight loss supplements, right? The before photo reveals some overweight, pale guy with scraggly hair—someone who seemingly just let himself go. But after using the latest and greatest weight loss supplement, the after photo reveals a very tan gentleman with a new haircut and a chiseled physique. It all looks and sounds great, but do you know what some supplement manufacturers and their marketing consultants typically do to create these ads? They pay some bodybuilder or fitness professional to get fat! That's right, the after picture is really the before picture, if you can believe that. It's a well-known industry secret, and it really shouldn't surprise any of us. After all, marketing is king when it comes to the world of supplements.

ated with these ingredients, including increased blood pressure, heart rate, and respiratory rate. Another potential issue is that companies often combine several of these ingredients into one product and then sell it as an energy or health supplement. Even then, many of the products don't deliver much bang for their buck. Plus, we don't know how any of these stimulants will specifically affect you as an individual, let alone several of them combined. Despite the claims, your best bet is to pass on these ingredients and the products that contain them. Instead, focus on maximizing your training and nutrition, and speak to a registered dietitian or certified personal trainer about losing body fat in the safest and most effective way possible.

Nitric Oxide Products

It wasn't that long ago when nitric oxide (NO) products were being touted as the next big thing in sports nutrition. And if you look at the sales for these types of products today, you would think the supplement manufacturers succeeded in making this a reality. But do NO products really work? Unfortunately, the majority of the research can't back up the hefty claims regarding enhanced muscle recovery and improved body composition. In fact, some very prominent researchers in sports nutrition dub it the most over-hyped supplement of all time. Now that's a pretty bold statement. NO products are typically sold as pre- or post-workout formulas, often combining several ingredients—some of which have been proven to work well, and some that have not. Ultimately, any benefits derived from these products are usually due to the ingredients that have strong research behind them. As a result, it's probably best to avoid NO products and their high price tags. Talk to a personal trainer or sports dietitian to find out what ingredients or products may help you gain a competitive edge for your training.

Energy Boosters

Energy supplements have been one of the fastest-growing supplement categories in the last year or two. Unfortunately, these energy shots aren't all they're cracked up to be. The ingredients are fairly standard and include B vitamins and an "energy blend" that usually contains caffeine and a variety of amino acids or their derivatives. B vitamins are known to help release the energy from food via biochemical pathways, but they don't provide energy directly. And if you wanted to get a simple caffeine fix, you'd probably just grab a cup of coffee, right? There's really nothing special here. In the end, it's probably best to pass on these energy supplements. Just consume enough energy in the form of food, work out regularly (since the endorphins that are released in the brain provide an energy boost), and get plenty of sleep so that you aren't so tired in the first place.

Superfruit Juices

Most of these products are exotic fruit juices marketed as super antioxidants, which supposedly have beneficial effects on the body. Sadly, many of these claims come from distributors (regular folks with limited knowledge of the products) and the elaborate marketing materials developed by the companies themselves. Research is often touted, too, but most of the studies typically referenced have been done on a specific fruit or an extract of that fruit, not the actual juice being sold to you. Plus, many of the manufacturers add other juice concentrates as well, so you have no idea how much of the supposed active ingredients are actually in the final product. But let's not forget one of the biggest issues with these juices—the cost. Many of them sell for $20 to $35 *per bottle*, with a typical serving being only a few ounces per day. The high cost is usually attributed to highly paid consultants and the distribution network itself, since everyone involved gets a piece of the monetary pie. The bottom line: These juices don't appear to be harmful, but are they actually making you any healthier? That question is hard to answer, but I'll go out on a limb and say probably not. For now, it's best to stick with your morning glass of good ol' orange juice!

A "WEIGHTY" ISSUE

Chris Farley uttered a seemingly obvious quip in *Tommy Boy*: "I have what doctors call a little bit of a weight problem." In the movie, it was a funny line by a funny guy, but sadly, this is the reality for far too many people nowadays. In all seriousness, the numbers haven't changed much. Sixty-eight percent of adults over age twenty are considered either overweight or obese.[1] That's roughly 150 million people in the United States alone! And yes, you read that correctly. But it's not just an adult problem, anymore. Overweight and obesity continue to rise in our younger generations, too. How did we get here? Why haven't our solutions worked up to this point? What do we do now? Let's try to answer these questions, because if we don't, things are only going to get worse (and frankly, that's hard to imagine).

CALORIES IN VERSUS CALORIES OUT: A HISTORY LESSON
So what happened—how did we get here? Most people would probably assume that as a result of all of the high-calorie convenience foods we cram into our fast-food lifestyles, we simply ate way more calories than our bodies needed, and we gained weight as a result. Seems logical, and with literally thousands of gluttonous examples to point to, you'd be hard-pressed to find fault with this conclusion. In fact, several researchers support this theory and often point

out that leisure-time activity has remained stable over the past few decades. Therefore, it must be calories in, right?

Well, other well-known scientists aren't quite as convinced. Some of them argue that calorie consumption hasn't increased nearly enough to account for the dramatic increase in overweight and obesity. Others find fault with the whole leisure-time activity theory, suggesting that there's something else at play here. As a result, a few of these nonconformists decided to study something that they thought would have an even more important impact on weight management—occupational physical activity. After all, time spent at work represents more total hours of the week than leisure-time activity, at least for most folks. These rogue researchers decided to analyze energy expenditure data from 1960 to 2008 from the U.S. Bureau of Labor Statistics and compared that with average body weights from the U.S. Health and Nutrition Examination Surveys. The findings were quite remarkable. The *daily* occupational energy expenditure dropped by 140 calories for men and was slightly less for women. But here's the amazing thing. The researchers found that this drop in expenditure accounted for almost all of the expected weight gain one might see from 1960 to 2003–2006. They also point out that in 1960, almost half of all private-sector jobs required at least moderate-intensity physical activity, but that this number decreased to below 20 percent in 2008.[2]

You're probably wondering why I decided to highlight this study. First of all, it's the first study of its kind, and it revealed some truly eye-opening results. Second, it's important to look at all aspects of an issue, especially one as important as the obesity epidemic. Accepting conventional

Q: Is detoxing appropriate for weight loss?

A: No. Detox diets might be popular right now, but they are definitely not the answer. Unfortunately, a lot of people think detoxification is a reasonable path to better health. So-called experts claim that detox diets can flush toxins from your body, strengthen your immune system, improve your skin, and help you get rid of excess fat fast. They even point to famous Hollywood starlets who, as we all know, are willing to try anything and everything to get "the look." Thankfully, most real experts, including doctors, dietitians, and trainers, agree that these regimens do more harm than good, often resulting in unpleasant, and sometimes dangerous, side effects. These side effects can include vitamin deficiencies, electrolyte abnormalities, blood sugar problems, diarrhea, muscle breakdown, and a suppressed immune system. Hopefully, it's not a surprise to you, but your body is perfectly capable of detoxifying itself, and it does an excellent job. Your kidneys, liver, lungs, skin, and several other organs all contribute to this process.

wisdom is never a good idea in the scientific world. And finally, this study helps to explain how we ended up being fatter than we've ever been. If we add these new findings to the existing body of research, it's reasonable to assume that some people have gained weight because they ate too much, others gained weight because they were too sedentary (apparently at work, if this study is any indication), and *most* gained weight because of some combination of the two. We can let the researchers continue to debate about which variable is more important, but clearly, we have a *huge* problem on our hands.

TRIMMING THE (DIETARY) FAT

If either increased caloric intake or decreased caloric expenditure—or more likely both—account for the obesity epidemic, then it seems that we should have been able to make a dent in this trend in the last few decades. Unfortunately, we have not. Nutritionally speaking, we've tried it all. In the 1980s and 1990s, we started with the low-fat craze, which seemed logical at the time, since fat has twice as many calories per gram compared with carbohydrates and proteins. So if you decreased your fat intake, you'd automatically decrease your calories, right? Sounds good, but in practice, this didn't happen. Most folks simply moved their caloric intake to carbohydrates. And as we all know, it's incredibly easy to over eat carbs. How many times have you craved a few pretzels or crackers, only to finish the entire box as you're lounging on the couch? Yeah, I've been there too. To coincide with this low-fat movement, the corporate food giants started creating all kinds of low-fat, fat-free, and low-calorie versions of some of their most popular products. Diet foods were going to be our savior, but moderation became an afterthought, and people ate way too much of this supposed health food. Fat-free cookies, low-fat muffins, and reduced-fat chips were all on the menu, yet the nation's waistline continued to bulge. Fat intake dropped, but carbohydrate intake skyrocketed, resulting in an increase in total calories for many. Clearly, this wasn't the answer we were looking for.

IT'S GOTTA BE THE CARBS

As the new millennium slowly approached, people saw that low-fat diets were ineffective at battling the bulge. Or was it that people weren't following what is considered a healthy

low-fat diet? After all, these diets should have worked well
(and they do work well, when followed properly), but when
you substitute *some* dietary fat for *a lot* of carbohydrate,
your success rate is gonna suck. You can guess what happened next. We had a new enemy in our midst—carbs! People cut out sodas and chips and crackers and doughnuts and
almost anything else that has even a morsel of carbohydrate. Even bread, rice, cereals, and pasta were on the chop-
ping block, and almost all fruit and even some vegetables
were taboo, too. Sure, lots of people lost a lot of weight, but
there were also noticeable side effects to following these
types of diets, and consumers really didn't stop to think
about the long-term implications. Was this type of dieting
healthy, and could it be maintained?

The healthfulness of the low-carb lifestyle is still de-
bated to this day, with several high-profile scientists claim-
ing that the concerns about health risks are overblown.
Others argue that the limits on carbohydrates are simply
unnecessary (especially for weight loss), and that the lack
of fiber, vitamins, minerals, and antioxidants is concerning,
to say the least. As with most popular regimens, the low-
carb phenomenon faded over time, not because of a lack of
success, but because people found the lifestyle too difficult
to follow in the long term. Interestingly, low-carb diets were
gradually replaced by "smart carb" plans based on the
glycemic index. The principles of the glycemic index are
somewhat complex, but suffice it to say, these diets provided even more carbohydrate confusion for consumers.
Both types of programs ended up being more fad than
lifestyle change, and most of the weight loss benefits were
short-lived.

FAD DIETS = WEIGHT LOSS SUCCESS?

Remember the cabbage soup diet or the blood-type diet or the grapefruit diet or the forty-eight-hour diet? Or have you heard of the hCG diet, which spotlights the use of a pregnancy hormone for both women *and* men? No matter how ridiculous any of these may seem, you can always find at least a few folks who have tried them. And you know what the funny thing is? The dieters were probably successful at losing weight. Although I hear quite often from both health professionals and consumers alike that fad diets don't work, most fad diets do indeed work, and some of them quite well. Let's face it—if the latest fad diet didn't elicit some sort of weight loss, it clearly wouldn't survive out on the market for very long. The problem is that almost every fad diet is a short-term solution to a long-term problem. These diets also tend to associate weight loss success with some gimmick when, in actuality, decreased calorie intake is usually the real reason for shedding the pounds. There's no mystery here. This is true of almost every diet out there.

SEARCHING FOR THE SILVER BULLET

We've all seen people successfully lose weight when they follow a particular program, but for some reason, that weight always seems to come back. We can safely sum up these diet failures in three problematic scenarios. The first is that most diet plans are too restrictive in one way or another. Either there aren't enough calories, carbohydrates (or fats), or solid food; these deficits end up leaving people feeling unsatisfied and yearning for more of what's missing. Plus, if you're getting too little of one thing, you're probably getting too much of another. Clearly, this is not the way to achieve variety, balance, and moderation in your eating plan. Another potential problem is a general lack of monitoring. If you're not paying strict attention to how much you're eating, you'll find it increasingly difficult to be successful. Research has proven this time and time again, but monitoring your progress takes extra work, and many people never commit the time or energy needed to keep track of their habits. The last issue, and probably one of the most obvious, is that people always seem to be looking for a quick fix. They simply aren't interested or haven't fully committed to changing their behaviors *permanently*. That's why fad diets gain so much popularity so quickly before fizzling out. They provide instant gratification, and that's something that our society yearns for more than anything else. But the weight loss is usually temporary, which means you'll probably be back in the same boat—or an even larger one—in the very near future.

MARRY NUTRITION, AND LET EXERCISE BE YOUR MISTRESS

We've seemingly tried it all when it comes to nutrition and weight loss, but can the same be said for exercise? In other words, maybe exercise is really the more important factor here, and our attention to nutrition has simply been misplaced over the last few decades. Is it possible that exercise has been the key to weight loss all along, and we were too clueless to realize it?

Thankfully, this isn't the case. Exercise is important for a variety of reasons and should always be discussed when you are devising a plan for weight loss. However, common sense suggests that nutrition is the more important variable, and here's why: If you've ever looked at food labels and compared them with the calorie counters on your exercise

> **DID YOU KNOW?**
>
> Yo-yo dieting—losing weight and then gaining it back multiple times—isn't as detrimental as we once thought. In the past, this practice was thought to have adverse consequences on body composition, metabolic rate, future weight loss attempts, and other health matters. But recent research hasn't necessarily found this to be the case. In fact, the National Task Force on the Prevention and Treatment of Obesity found that weight cycling had no adverse effects on metabolism, body composition, risk factors for cardiovascular disease, or on future weight loss efforts.[3] So just because you've failed to keep weight off in the past doesn't mean you shouldn't try again. However, it's important to make lifestyle changes you can stick with so you don't end up in a continuous pattern of weight cycling.

equipment, you're likely to come to some startling conclusions. It is much easier to decrease your calorie intake by 300 to 500 calories per day than it is to expend that many more calories each day through exercise.

Unfortunately, traditional strength training doesn't burn all that many calories, and neither does stretching. Cardiovascular exercise can burn a significant amount of calories, but only if you increase either the intensity or the duration of exercise, or both. But even if you exercise at a relatively high intensity for an hour or two a day, it's too easy to negate that calorie burn by stuffing your face with food or sucking down calorie-laden beverages. (See our examples in "The Energy Cost of Food" sidebar if you want some proof.) Plus, who works out for an hour or two every day, anyway? The trend is toward shorter, more efficient workouts. And if this

THE ENERGY COST OF FOOD

When I said the calories burned via exercise are easily ne-
gated by calories consumed via foods and beverages, I wasn't
kidding around. It's a real eye-opener! Let's see how much
exercise a guy my size (154 pounds) would have to do to burn
the same amount of calories found in some common, everyday foods and beverages.

- To burn off one 8-ounce glass of skim milk, I'd have to
  walk briskly (3.5 mph) for 20 minutes.
- To burn off one 6-ounce Yoplait Light yogurt, I'd have to
  do gardening for about 20 minutes.
- To burn off one chewy granola bar, I'd have to rake the
  lawn for 30 minutes.
- To burn off one cup of grapes, I'd have to do yoga for
  35 minutes.
- To burn off one McDonald's hamburger, I'd have to
  punch the heavy bag for 35 minutes.
- To burn off two slices of Pizza Hut supreme pizza,
  I'd have to use the elliptical at a moderate pace for
  60 minutes.
- To burn off a Starbucks caffé mocha with whole milk,
  I'd have to do strength training for almost 90 minutes.
- To burn off one cup of Ben & Jerry's New York Super
  Fudge Chunk, I'd have to shovel snow for 90 minutes.

As you can see, we're definitely fighting an uphill battle
when it comes to calories in versus calories out. Thankfully,
our bodies burn quite a few calories just to keep us alive and
well. After that, the onus is on you to be as active as you can
be, both through leisure-time activity and exercise, so that
you can enjoy some of the foods you like while still reaching
your weight goals.

is the case, then maybe your nonexercise activity is important since it makes up such a significant portion of your day. The occupational physical activity study that we mentioned earlier was alluding to this very point. We'll discuss all of these issues in the exercise chapters in Part 4.

Let me be clear. Exercise is certainly beneficial for overall health, and it can help move the needle in the right direction from a weight management perspective, but *only* if the nutrition side of the equation is under control. Think of it like this: It is relatively easy to lose weight by simply watching what you eat, even without exercise. Many people have tried this and found success. But try to do the same with exercise only, and you'll find it to be almost impossible.

THE TRUE BENEFIT OF EXERCISE

What scientists and consumers have discovered is that exercise plays a much more prominent role in weight maintenance after you have successfully lost weight. To see this point, you can look to the National Weight Control Registry. The registry is the largest prospective study investigating weight loss maintenance. The sole focus has been to identify the characteristics of people who have lost weight and kept it off long term. The researchers are currently following more than five thousand people, and at this point, the participants have lost an average of 66 pounds and have kept it off for 5½ years! Interestingly, exercise seems to play a very big role. On average, about 90 percent of the registry participants exercise for an hour a day.[4] This is no small feat, and the take-home message is clear. If you want to maintain a significant weight loss, you'd better be prepared to move.

GIMME THE NUTRITIONAL GAME PLAN

In some ways, this is a diet book, and so you want to see the diet, right? You might be wondering if we recommend a particular nutritional philosophy. In other words, do we recommend one universal, optimal diet that helps everyone lose those 1 to 2 pounds per week? The answer is no; there is no one-size-fits-all approach to weight management and general health—various plans work for different people. But regardless of which plan you choose, it should meet the following three criteria:

- It gets you to your desired weight, assuming you have one.
- It promotes health and helps prevent chronic disease.
- It is sustainable for the long term.

Another important point needs to be stressed here as well. Eating for health and eating for weight loss are really one and the same. In fact, you should follow similar nutritional guidelines if you're looking to gain weight, too, though there may be a few minor exceptions. Regardless of what your weight management goal might be, you should always strive to accomplish that goal in the healthiest way possible.

THE GOVERNMENT GOT IT RIGHT (FOR THE MOST PART)

OK, now that we've got that covered, it's time for some specifics. It's obvious that we should eat more of the right stuff, less of the wrong stuff, move more during our daily activities, and try to exercise as often as we can. Though these recommendations fall in line with my "Keep it simple, Stupid" philosophy, we clearly need to go even further. Ironically enough, the U.S. government's 2010 Dietary Guidelines for Americans offer a nice summary of dos and don'ts when it comes to nutrition and physical activity. They're a good starting point, but be prepared to modify them to fit your particular lifestyle. Check out the complete list below, and try to identify areas where you could improve.[1]

- Control total calorie intake to manage body weight. For people who are overweight or obese, this will mean consuming fewer calories from foods and beverages.
- Increase physical activity, and reduce time spent in sedentary behaviors.
- Reduce daily sodium intake to less than 2,300 milligrams (mg), and further reduce intake to 1,500 mg among persons who are fifty-one and older and those of any age who are African American or have hypertension, diabetes, or chronic kidney disease.
- Consume less than 10 percent of calories from saturated fatty acids by replacing them with monounsaturated and polyunsaturated fatty acids.
- Consume less than 300 mg of dietary cholesterol per day.
- Keep trans fatty acid consumption as low as possible by limiting foods that contain synthetic sources of trans

fats, such as partially hydrogenated oils, and by limiting other solid fats.

- Reduce the intake of calories from solid fats and added sugars.
- Limit the consumption of foods that contain refined grains, especially refined grain foods that contain solid fats, added sugars, and sodium.
- If alcohol is consumed, it should be consumed in moderation—up to one drink per day for women and two drinks per day for men—and only by adults of legal drinking age.

If you're striving to be healthy, you should meet the following recommendations while staying within your calorie needs.

- Increase vegetable and fruit intake.
- Eat a variety of vegetables, especially dark-green and red and orange vegetables and beans and peas.
- Consume at least half of all grains as whole grains. Increase whole-grain intake by replacing refined grains with whole grains.
- Increase intake of fat-free or low-fat milk and other dairy products, such as yogurt and cheese, and fortified soy beverages.
- Choose a variety of protein foods, which include seafood, lean meat and poultry, eggs, beans and peas, soy products, and unsalted nuts and seeds.
- Increase the amount and variety of seafood consumed by choosing seafood in place of some meat and poultry.
- Replace protein foods that are higher in solid fats with choices that are lower in solid fats and calories or that

DID YOU KNOW?

Fast food doesn't necessarily need to be avoided if weight loss is your goal. We all know it isn't the healthiest meal in town, but we also know that being realistic is an important component of any successful weight loss program. Let's face it, if you're crunched for time, fast food may be your only reasonable option—for an occasional trip, not four or five weekly trips. The same principle applies for sit-down restaurants as well. It's just way too easy to deviate from your nutrition plan when you're eating away from home. Aim for no more than two meals out each week, and be sure to make healthy, commonsense choices whenever possible. The key is to watch out for calorie-laden foods with added sugars, sodium, and fat, and control your portions as much as possible. Look for the Nutrition Facts pamphlets in your local restaurants or on their Web sites, and educate yourself on the menus. If you make the effort, you'll be able to find a sensible meal, no matter where you go. Remember, balance, variety, and moderation are the words to live by when it comes to food. If you apply these principles regularly, you won't have to sacrifice your health and wellness goals when eating out.

are sources of oils. In other words, moderate your consumption of meat, poultry, and eggs, and increase your consumption of seafood, nuts, and seeds.

- Use oils to replace solid fats where possible.
- Choose foods that provide more potassium, dietary fiber, calcium, and vitamin D, all of which are nutrients of concern in American diets. These foods include vegetables, fruits, whole grains, and milk and milk products.

This list is long, but it's not quantum physics. Most of us know we should increase our fruit and vegetable intake, cut down on things like sodium, trans fats, and added sugars, and limit our alcohol consumption as much as possible. Personally, I think we should try to eat a few more vegetarian meals as well, though you don't see this recommendation listed above. None of these ideas are new, yet we seem to fail at putting them into practice, at least on a consistent basis.

If you do struggle to put these guidelines into practice, the U.S. Department of Agriculture is here to help. In 2011, it put out a simple new guide to help consumers make healthy choices at mealtimes. Called MyPlate, the guideline replaces the old MyPyramid that caused so much confusion for so many. The MyPlate graphic depicts one-quarter of the plate as grains, one-quarter as protein, one-quarter as vegetables, and one-quarter as fruit, with a serving of dairy on the side. The guide is very user-friendly and gives people easy-to-follow recommendations, though I would have made one obvious change. Why not make half the plate vegetables, as most dietitians suggest anyway, and then add fruit as a side serving, similar to the dairy? Regardless, the plate graphic already has a lot of support among scientists and consumers. Ultimately, people who are able to follow the Dietary Guidelines and plan meals according to MyPlate will end up healthier in all aspects of life. If you'd like more information on either of these resources, check out http://www.choosemyplate.gov/

BULK IS BETTER
In addition to the guidelines presented above, there's one other important nutritional concept that should be applied

CHECK THIS OUT!

When people are looking for snack options, convenience always seems to trump everything, and nutrition ends up taking a backseat. But look no further. Give some of these nutritious options a try. You'll be glad you did!

Celery and carrots with low-fat dip
Plain yogurt with granola and blueberries
Whole-grain crackers with hummus
Cottage cheese with apple slices
Trail mix with dried fruit and nuts
String cheese and a banana
½ whole-grain bagel with peanut butter
Popcorn
Rice cakes with lean ham or turkey
Edamame (soybeans in the pod)

on a daily basis, especially if weight management is a concern. It's something I've used with my own clients for years, and it works well in both the research lab and the real world. The concept involves two components of the diet—water and fiber—which have recently been touted for their weight-loss-enhancing effects. Why? Because they help to lower the energy density of a food, which is defined as the number of calories in a given amount (often expressed in calories per gram). This approach has garnered attention because of research conducted by Barbara Rolls, a Penn State University professor, on satiety (fullness). She discovered that fiber and water add "bulk" to food without increasing the calorie load much at all. Therefore, if you consume foods that have more

fiber and water and that are subsequently lower in energy
density, you'll be able to eat more food for fewer calories.
Rolls dubbed the concept *volumetrics*.

Dieters often complain of feeling deprived, so Rolls may
be onto something here. Who wouldn't want the ability to

Q: How many calories does a person need to eat to lose
weight?

A: It would be easy to say that the average female should take
in about 1,200 to 1,500 calories to lose weight, and males
should shoot for 1,800 to 2,100, but that doesn't mean that
these numbers will necessarily work for you. The ability to
lose weight depends on a number of variables, most notably
your resting metabolic rate and your activity level (both general daily activities and exercise). These factor into the expenditure side of the energy balance equation, which then
helps to determine the intake side as well. Let's see how many
calories I should eat if I wanted to lose approximately one
pound per week:

- Resting metabolic rate (based on my weight of 154
  pounds, my height of five feet ten, and my age of thirty-
  five): 1,641 calories
- Add 20 percent (328 calories) for general daily activities,
  excluding exercise: 1,969 calories
- Add 350 calories for exercise each day: 2,319 calories
- Subtract 500 calories to elicit a one pound weight loss
  per week: **1,819** calories
- If you're interested in calculating your own calorie
  needs, check out www.anytimehealth.com.

eat more food while losing unwanted weight or maintaining their current weight? And the great thing about applying this energy density principle is the fact that the foods we chronically under-eat are the lowest in terms of energy density, so it encourages us to consume the stuff we should be eating, anyway. I'm talking about fruits, vegetables, whole grains, and even things like broth-based soups. In the end, weight management is achieved and overall nutrition improves as well.

CARBS, AND PROTEINS, AND FATS, OH, MY!

One last issue often puzzles folks, and it involves the macronutrients—carbohydrates, proteins, and fats. Because of all the varying nutritional philosophies out there, people can get confused about how much of each macronutrient they should take in or what percentage of their calories each should comprise. And everyone seems to do something different. Some advocate higher carb; some, higher protein; and some, very low fat. In truth, it really depends on your goals. As discussed earlier, there are acceptable macronutrient distribution ranges (AMDRs) that we can use as guides. Generally speaking, you should shoot for 45 to 65 percent carbohydrate, 10 to 35 percent protein, and 20 to 35 percent fat. If you're an athlete or you're focused on the cardio end of the exercise spectrum, then you should be more liberal with your carb intake. If you're focused on strength training and you're looking to add mass and size, you'd be wise to aim for approximately 50 percent carbohydrate, 25 percent protein, and 25 percent fat. If you're like most folks and could benefit from dropping a few pounds, it may be advisable to stay on the lower end of the carbohydrate range.

Then, divvy up the rest of your calories between healthy proteins and fats. Remember, these percentage changes may not seem like much, but there's usually varying calorie levels associated with each of these goals.

Following these general recommendations is a good start, but it's also in your best interest to individualize as needed. If you are interested in following a calorie-controlled meal plan that incorporates the nutritional philosophy detailed in this chapter, be sure to check out the 21-day plan at the end of the book.

TRACKING AND SUCCESS GO HAND IN HAND

It's amazing how clueless people seem to be when it comes to estimating the number of calories they should consume in a given day. In fact, an online survey conducted by *USA Today* in July 2010 indicated that "63% couldn't accurately estimate the number, 25% wouldn't even venture a guess, and only 12% can nail it."[2] No wonder people have such a hard time managing their weight.

There is a solution to this dilemma. First of all, it's important to determine your daily calorie needs. This includes your resting metabolic rate, calories burned through daily activities and exercise, and then additional calorie adjustments based on your particular weight goals. Guessing is not an option here, and luckily, there are plenty of Web sites that can help you determine your specific number (check out www.anytimehealth.com for more information).

Once you know your calorie needs, monitoring becomes essential. If you truly want to control your weight, nothing could be more important than tracking your food intake. As a registered dietitian with many years' experience in helping people get healthy, I can tell you that the great majority of my clients were successful when they recorded their food intake, even if only for a few days every couple months. Plus, it's so easy to do these days with the all the health and wellness Web sites and smartphone apps available. There's really no excuse not to, especially if you're new to the weight loss game or you're stuck in a plateau. The bottom line: The more information you gather about your own health and wellness habits, the easier it will be to achieve your goals.

Monitoring your intake is crucial, but here are a few other tips that will keep you on track nutritionally.

- Pay attention to appetite versus hunger. Appetite is the psychological need for food, but hunger is physiological. You feel hunger in your stomach when your body needs food, so don't ignore it.
- Avoid skipping meals. Keeping a consistent energy level throughout the day can be difficult, especially if you ignore mealtimes.
- Don't grocery shop on an empty stomach. You'll end up buying food you didn't intend to, and you'll probably buy more than you need.
- Plan out a week's worth of meals, and do most of the prep work at the beginning of the week. We all get time-crunched, which can make you make bad choices about food if you aren't prepared.

PART 4

FITNESS SUCKS, TOO, BUT . . .

OK, I'm sure you see the logic here. If both changing your behaviors and eating well kinda suck, despite being important for long-term health and wellness, then working out shouldn't be any different, right? After all, it takes physical effort—actual energy—to move around, and lying on the couch is easier and probably more comfortable. But how do you feel after lying on said couch in the same position for two or three hours, after watching one of those ridiculously long *Lord of the Rings* movies, for example? What does it feel like to make those first few movements? I'm guessing you feel a little stiff, maybe a little sore, and you're probably regretting the lack of activity that was your life for the past few hours. So if this is how you feel after being inactive for far too long, and it holds true for both fit and unfit folks (and I assure you, it does), then maybe you and the rest of us should be inactive for shorter periods. Novel idea, I know!

This is the essence of the fitness section. Let's move a little more so we feel better. Or maybe it's so that we don't feel worse. Whatever it is, movement is what we are meant to do, and sadly, our environments require us to do less and less. So let's start moving more frequently and more effectively for both fitness and health. And if you're busy, like most people I know, we'll figure out a way for you to get in quality *exercise* in a lot less time. Are you prepared for a fact-finding, myth-busting expedition into the world of fitness? Let's go . . .

MOVING IS NEAT

Park further away from the building. Take the stairs instead of the elevator. You've heard these phrases numerous times, and you've probably done one or the other at some point in the past. Still, have you ever stopped to think about how beneficial taking the stairs instead of the elevator could be for your health? The basic premise here is that doing just a little extra activity is good for you. This shouldn't be surprising.

A NEW IDEA BUBBLES UP

But what if I told you that not doing it is actually detrimental to health? What if I told you that our collective inactivity has fostered an entire area of study called inactivity physiology? And what if I told you experts have already concluded that too much sitting is *not* the same as too little activity? In other words, too much sitting has its own independent health risks, regardless of your physical activity level. Many scientists actually believe that our country's severe lack of general daily activity (non-exercise activity) has been a significant causal factor in the overweight and obesity epidemic. The bottom line—none of this is good news!

JAMES LEVINE TO THE RESCUE

James Levine, a world-renowned obesity researcher and physician from the Mayo Clinic in Rochester, Minnesota, has been studying something called non-exercise activity thermogenesis (NEAT) for years. NEAT is essentially the energy we expend when we're not eating, sleeping, or exercising. It's the calories we burn when we're not thinking about burning calories, and it contributes about 15 percent to the total daily energy expenditure in sedentary individuals and as much as 50 percent in very active folks. Unfortunately, with desk jobs, TV watching, and Web surfing now the norm, the calories expended during general daily tasks has diminished greatly. Some researchers actually believe that the movement (pardon the pun) from a manual-labor-based workforce to a desk-centric one has been the biggest factor in the obesity epidemic. We discussed some of this research in the weight management chapter. Other researchers, including Levine, point out that our collective calorie intake hasn't increased much at all in recent decades, or at least not enough to account for the huge rise in overweight and obesity. They believe this to be true, despite the prevalence of things like french fries, potato chips, soda, and other high-calorie foods and beverages. Therefore, maybe non-exercise activity is the real culprit here.

In 2005, Levine published some interesting research that centered on the concept of NEAT. He monitored the activity of twenty individuals and found that the lean participants were on their feet for two more hours each day compared with the obese folks. This amounted to an additional 350 calories burned per day, which could account for a thirty- to forty-pound weight loss in a year.[1] These very impressive numbers speak to the importance of simply moving more, even without exercise. Unfortunately, people's environments are simply too conducive to sedentary lifestyles, so change really needs to start there. If your environment is one in which activity is encouraged and inactivity is discouraged, good things are bound to happen.

TRACKING NEAT

The best thing about this area of study is that we now have technological devices that can track NEAT. After all, if your goal is to consistently move more each day, it certainly helps to know where you're starting from. And having access to your daily calorie burn is a strong motivating factor to continue that movement. There are numerous accelerometer-based devices on the market, and many of them work quite well. Most of them sync up with an online platform and generally cost around $100, though some may be a bit more expensive.

SO WHERE DO WE GO FROM HERE?

The great thing is that improving your NEAT is much easier than you might think. I'm not talking about going to the gym to throw around the weights or going on a five-mile run. We'll focus on these aspects of fitness in the coming chapters. What I am talking about is simply *sitting less*, which equates to moving more. That means doing almost anything, because, frankly, anything is better than nothing. Start incorporating some of these basic activities into your daily routine, with the goal of making them habits.

- Yes, whenever possible, park further away from your destination.
- And yep, take the stairs instead of the elevator.
- Disconnect from the Internet after 8 p.m. (or earlier) each night.

- Keep the TV off for at least two hours when you get home in the evening.
- Break up your day by taking three 10-minute walks— morning, lunch, and afternoon.
- Play with your kids or your pets for at least an hour each evening.

If you can make these very simple activities stick over the coming weeks and months, you'll feel better, look better, and be healthier. And then you can start to find new ways of incorporating activity into your life.

THE CARDIO PRESCRIPTION

From an exercise perspective, cardiovascular exercise should definitely be front and center. *Cardiovascular* essentially means the types of exercise that increase your heart rate. After all, your heart is the single most important muscle in your entire body. And if working your muscles is beneficial to muscular health, then it stands to reason that working your heart would be good for heart health. In fact, cardiovascular exercise produces several beneficial changes. These include improvements in blood pressure, glucose tolerance, insulin sensitivity, blood lipid levels, and inflammatory markers.[1] In other words, it's just good for you, plain and simple.

THE GO-TO FORM OF EXERCISE
Times certainly have changed, though. As people gravitate toward shorter and more-efficient workouts, is traditional cardio (20 to 45 minutes on the treadmill, elliptical, or bike) becoming a thing of the past? Not necessarily. The various types of workouts simply give people more options, and when it comes to exercise, the more options you have, the more inclined you'll be to stick with your program. And since our focus is on beginners, traditional cardiovascular exercise becomes even more important, since most folks start off with fairly basic cardio sessions and gradually

progress to more-advanced workouts as their fitness levels improve.

Let's briefly review the FITT principles (frequency, intensity, type, and time) for cardiovascular exercise, and then discuss a few nontraditional ways to get your workouts in. We'll also focus on a few common misconceptions surrounding this particular form of exercise. After that, you'll be ready to get started.

WHAT'S A GUY OR GAL TO DO?

If cardio is so important to overall health and fitness, a logical question might be, what type of cardio exercise should I do? What would you say if I told you it really doesn't matter? You can do almost any form of exercise that gets your heart rate up, and you'll reap the benefits. If you're a total newbie, things like walking, jogging, and even playing yard games with your kids all work quite well. And if you've just

Q: What should I do first—cardio or strength training?

A: This is an ongoing debate. Some might say that you should do cardio first because it's a nice way to warm up your muscles before a weight-training session. Others would argue that doing cardio first will cause too much fatigue, which might lower your workout intensity and make lifting with proper form more difficult. There really isn't a right or wrong answer. The best advice is to pay attention to your goals. And if you're new to exercise, simply do your lifting and cardio on opposite days, since you'll probably be doing only two to three sessions of each for the first few weeks, anyway.

CHECK THIS OUT!

Before you get into the meat of your cardio session, it's important to do a short warm-up. Unfortunately, most people simply don't make time for it. Lots of folks just want to get in and get out—understandable, as we're all busy and it's enough sometimes to even find time for a workout. But there are benefits to properly preparing the body for exercise. Warming up

increases the temperature of your muscles and joints, which makes movement more efficient and reduces the risk of injury;

causes blood vessels to dilate, which shuttles oxygen and nutrients to the muscles; and

prepares you for exercise mentally, allowing you to focus on the work at hand.

In the end, you will feel better and perform better if you include a warm-up in your exercise session. Take five minutes, and do some light cardio—try the elliptical machine or some fast walking—along with a few basic strengthening exercises, such as lunges, push-ups, squats, or planks, which use your own body weight. And don't forget to do a nice 5-minute cooldown at the end to gradually lower your heart rate.

started going to the gym, you're likely to be using one of the more traditional pieces of cardio equipment: the treadmill, bike, elliptical, or rower. Again, these are great forms of exercise that produce similar results from the cardiovascular perspective. The most important thing is to find something (or a few things) that you enjoy doing, and then stick with them. And as your fitness level improves, you can increase the duration or intensity of your workouts or move on to new and more challenging exercises.

One other thing to consider as you start a cardio program is the importance of cross-training. In cross-training, you find a few types of exercise that you enjoy, and then rotate them consistently so that your body doesn't get used to the same thing. Eating a monotonous diet isn't a good idea, and neither is following a monotonous exercise program. Cross-training allows you to condition the entire body, add more flexibility to your workouts, and suffer fewer (or completely avoid) overuse injuries. Plus, it just makes working out more fun because you're always doing something new. Interestingly, there really aren't any specific guidelines to follow. In other words, if you like walking, playing tag with your kids, and the occasional game of golf or tennis, then just consistently mix these forms of exercise. Remember, boredom is one of the biggest reasons people stop exercising. Cross-training is just one way to prevent boredom from setting in from the get-go.

HOW MUCH AND HOW OFTEN?

According to the *2008 Physical Activity Guidelines for Americans*, adults should shoot for 150 minutes of moderate-intensity aerobic activity or 75 minutes of vigorous-intensity activity, ideally spread throughout an entire week. And doubling these numbers provides even greater health benefits.[2] Regardless of these recommendations, what you really have to do is factor in personal variables, like your current fitness level and your schedule. In other words, if you're completely new to exercise, it's certainly reasonable to start out with 20 to 30 minutes two to three times per week. And if you can't do that, start with whatever you can do, whether it's 2 minutes, 5 minutes, or 10 minutes. Even if you have an incredibly busy schedule, fitting in two 10-minute walks each day will get you very close to the preceding recommendation over a seven-day period. As your fitness level improves and you become more comfortable with exercise, you can start incorporating additional workout days. It's not uncommon for advanced exercisers to do cardio four, five, or even six days a week, depending on their fitness goals.

THE INTENSITY CAN MAKE ALL THE DIFFERENCE

The last issue that needs to be addressed is the intensity of your cardio sessions. Again, since we're focusing on beginners, your best bet is to use the talk test. This is an old method of determining an appropriate intensity level for

---

HIGH-INTENSITY INTERVAL TRAINING

If you've been working out for a while and have a sound fitness base, then high-intensity interval training might be for you. It's a fantastic way to work out, and it offers many of the same advantages of more traditional training programs in much less time. The idea is to pick an activity that you like to do, and then fluctuate between periods of high-intensity, sprint-type work and less intense, active recovery periods. This type of pattern is repeated several times until you've completed 15 to 20 minutes of work, not counting your warm-up and cool-down. The specific ratio you choose will depend primarily on your fitness level, but the goal is to finish the entire workout in about 30 minutes. If you're up for a challenge, give it a try!

exercise. Ideally, you should get to a level that makes it difficult to hold a conversation with someone while you're exercising. This doesn't mean you have to start a conversation
with the individual next to you, or that you can't exercise by
yourself. Just use your best judgment and make your workout challenging—just not so challenging that you can't complete the 10, 20, or 30 minutes that you set out to do.

As you start a cardio program, it's important to keep a
consistent pace rather than going really hard for a few minutes and then backing off because your body just can't keep
up. The latter practice—where you go all out for a short time
and then drop back to a more sustainable pace, and repeat
this pattern several times during a workout—is called *interval training*. Ideally, interval training is reserved for those
who have a solid fitness foundation to work from. In the
meantime, be sure to check out our beginner cardio sessions included in the 21-day fitness plan at the end of the
book.

IS STRENGTH THE
NEW CARDIO?

For years, the buzz in the fitness world revolved around cardiovascular exercise. Everyone seemed to do some form of cardio, and strength training took a backseat. Only the bodybuilding crowd really got into lifting weights. Gradually, this trend has changed. We now realize how beneficial strength training is, and because people are looking to do more efficient workouts, many workouts now combine strength and cardio in creative ways. In other words, the days of doing cardio all by itself are long gone.

DON'T CALL IT A COMEBACK

There must be a logical reason for the resurgence of strength training. And if you look at the benefits of doing this form of exercise, you'll begin to understand. Strength training reduces the risk of a number of chronic diseases and has been found to improve body composition, blood glucose levels, insulin sensitivity, and blood pressure. It also has a positive impact on bone and mental health. What's more, people typically report feeling more energized, which hopefully encourages that much more physical activity.[1] This list is pretty impressive, given that most people think weight training is simply about putting on more muscle mass. That's clearly part of the equation here, but more importantly, strength training is beneficial for long-term health. In the end, that's what truly matters.

I hope you're convinced that strength training is important enough to do on a consistent basis. If that's the case, let's provide some details regarding the FITT principles: frequency, intensity, type, and time.

STRENGTH RECOMMENDATIONS MADE EASY
When people think of strength training, dumbbells and barbells (free weights) come to mind. However, numerous types of strength training can be included in an exercise program. Machines, cables, bands, medicine balls, and even

CHECK THIS OUT!

Functional training has taken over. Things like TRX bands, Bosu balls, and stability balls are incredibly popular, and for good reason. They're new, innovative, and fun to use. But best of all, they're functional, which means that using them allows you to mimic traditional daily activities, thereby improving movement, balance, coordination, and strength all at the same time. That's pretty cool! The only real concern here is that people may not know how to use these pieces of equipment properly, which could potentially result in injury. There's definitely a learning curve with these products, so it's best to watch the experts first. I also strongly recommend working with a trainer until you're completely comfortable with the training methodology. As always, the goal is to educate yourself so you can get the most out of whatever training you decide to do.

body-weight exercises can all increase muscular strength and endurance. Even yoga can increase strength, and if you've tried it, you know what I'm talking about. And the best part is that many of these exercises can be performed at home. With so many options available to you, it's best to change up your workouts as often as possible. There's an entire library of exercise videos available on www.anytime health.com, so if you're interested in starting a strength-training program or you're looking to add something new to your existing program, then be sure to check them out. You can also ask a personal trainer to show you how to safely add some of these training methods to your workouts using proper technique and form.

One important issue that shouldn't be ignored is the idea of creating balance within your workouts. You obviously want to work all the major muscle groups, which include the following: chest, back, shoulders, arms, legs, and core (the abdominals, obliques, and low back). Having balanced workouts will create a balanced body, which is essentially what we all strive for when strength training.

HOW MUCH IS ENOUGH?

The frequency of strength training can range from two days per week for beginners to five or even six days per week for more advanced folks, though it also depends on your goals. If you're a newbie or you're concerned about simply main-taining your current level of muscle tissue, two to three whole-body circuit sessions per week is certainly enough. However, if you're really looking to add mass and size, then doing split routines (working different muscles on different days) several days a week may be more appropriate. It's also

Q: Are muscular imbalances a common problem when strength training?

A: They certainly can be for people just starting out. Most of us have a dominant side that becomes stronger as we age, thanks to repetitive use. This leaves us with a weaker side, which can make strength training a bit more challenging. Luckily, these weaknesses can be overcome. If you engage in a regular lifting program, your weaker side will gradually catch up over time. You don't even need to focus specifically on your weaker areas, though many people do in order to balance things out a bit faster. In the end, consistent training and time will create a balanced and strong body, so just stick with it!

important to make sure that you include two rest days for a particular muscle group before you decide to work it again.

When it comes to the number of sets you should perform, theories abound. Generally speaking, anywhere between two and ten seems appropriate per muscle group, though again, it depends on your fitness level. Obviously, we're focused on beginners, so staying on the low end (two to four sets per muscle group) will be enough to elicit significant gains in the first six to eight weeks of a program.

The intensity of the exercises is another factor to consider as well. Beginners should try to perform each exercise for eight to twelve repetitions, with the goal of completing one set within 45 to 60 seconds. And the goal would be to complete your entire strength-training workout in 30 to 45 minutes.

As you adapt to your program, you'll be able to increase the *volume* (defined as the number of sets multiplied by the number of repetitions, or reps) of your workouts, which will be likely to improve your results even more. If you need some guidance when it comes to strength training or you just want to know what to do for the first few weeks, check out our 21-day fitness plan at the end of the book.

THE MYTHS OF STRENGTH TRAINING

Pumping iron has been part of the fitness fabric for eons— as have a whole variety of strength-training myths. But here's the real deal . . .

MYTH 1: The calories you burn *after* a workout contribute significantly to your total daily energy expenditure.

It's true that you continue to burn calories even after finishing exercise, and the degree to which you burn those calories is largely dependent on the intensity and duration of that exercise. As a result, many people will tell you that strength training turns you into a calorie-burning machine for the next 24 to 48 hours afterward. Unfortunately, research has proven this isn't the case. The calories you burn after your workout do not contribute significantly to total daily energy expenditure.[2] What you need to be concerned with are the calories burned *during* your workout session. Then, just try to be more active throughout the rest of your day as well!

MYTH 2: You should follow the no-pain, no-gain philosophy when strength training.

Weight training sessions can be intense, resulting in microtears and subsequent muscle soreness for a day or two afterward. This is completely normal, and as the body heals

---

DID YOU KNOW?

Personal trainers can literally transform your life. They educate, motivate, and inspire, and frankly, that's worth its weight
in gold. From goal setting and proper exercise form to program design and diet advice, trainers have the answers. But
that's not even the best part. Trainers offer accountability,
friendship, and a much-needed support system as you embark on your wellness journey. Let's face it—we all struggle
with getting to the gym now and then. But trainers can make
working out a lot of fun, and they can challenge you consistently, which will ultimately get you better results. Look at it
this way . . . if your car needs to be fixed, you take it to a me-
chanic because he (or she!) has the expertise and skills to fix
your car. The same can be said for your body. Take care of it as
well as you can, and if you need help, seek out an expert at
your local club. Just make sure the person has solid creden-
tials and a strong background in fitness, kinesiology, strength
and conditioning, or sports medicine.

---

itself, the muscle fibers gradually become larger and
stronger. This is the essence of strength training. However, if
the implication here is that a workout is effective only if
pain is involved, that's simply untrue. Mild discomfort is
common at the end of a hard set as fatigue starts to set in,
but actual pain is never a good sign during a workout. If
you're experiencing this, it usually means you're severely
overworking a muscle or you've suffered an injury.

MYTH 3: You can work out when sick.

You often hear people say that working out is fine if it's
just a head cold—stuffy nose, coughing, and other stuff that

you don't like, but can deal with. This is probably OK, but if
you have a fever, body aches, or other more serious symp-
toms, you should leave the exercising to the rest of us. This
philosophy probably works for most of you, but here's my
take. When I'm working out, I don't really want people who
are sneezing and coughing around me—and you probably
don't, either. Plus, to work out with intensity, you should put
a premium on the *quality* of your exercise. Therefore, you're
better off resting up for a day or two, even if you just have a
head cold. Then, when you get back to exercising, you can
pick up right where you left off. I recommend you give it a
try. You might find it to be a good idea, and you'll keep the
germaphobes happy!

MYTH 4: Women will bulk up if they strength train.

It's *possible*, but unlikely. First of all, women simply don't
have the proper hormonal balance to put on huge amounts
of muscle tissue. Second, even if they did have the right
physiology, it would take some serious training to do it. Getting bigger muscles requires high-volume workouts (lots of
sets and reps) and a pretty high intensity as well. Picking up
a few weights here and there isn't a recipe for building
mass—it's what you do and how you do it that really makes
the difference. Strength-training programs can always be
tailored to specific goals, so if a woman doesn't want to put
on large amounts of muscle, that's just fine. Generally
speaking, a full-body circuit with higher rep ranges a few
days per week would work well for toning and the mainte-
nance of current muscle tissue.

STRETCH MUCH?

Despite being fairly athletic, I've never been all that flexible. It's unfortunate, too, since flexibility is a really important part of physical fitness. In fact, it's just as important as strength training and cardiovascular conditioning, though most folks don't adhere to a regular stretching program like they do with these other forms of exercise. I think it's about time we changed our attitude toward flexibility.

WHO KNEW STRETCHING WAS SO GOOD FOR YOU?

There are several forms of stretching, but the form you're probably most familiar with is static stretching, where you hold a particular position for a specific time. Most people perform this type, and that's completely fine. Generally speaking, the various forms of stretching all offer similar benefits, including the potential for injury prevention, an increased efficiency of movement, and improved blood flow and nutrient delivery to the joints. Stretching also improves muscle coordination, overall balance, and postural alignment. It can even help to alleviate muscle soreness and stress after a workout. Not bad for just a few minutes of relaxation! Unfortunately, these benefits aren't tangible to most folks; stretching doesn't give you bigger muscles, for instance. Because the benefits can't be seen or, in some cases, even felt, people end up skipping flexibility exercises altogether. Not an ideal situation if you're truly concerned about your overall fitness level.

MORE IS BETTER

Ideally, static stretches should be held for 15 to 30 seconds, with the goal of accruing 60 seconds per flexibility exercise. This means you may end up doing two to four reps for each stretch. The optimum routine should target the following areas: neck, chest, back, shoulders, core, hips, legs, and ankles. These exercises can be done as few as two days per week, but some people do them daily or at least after every workout. Either one is appropriate, but you may reap additional benefits if you stretch more often.

One question that often puzzles people is when to do their flexibility exercises. We all grew up with the notion that stretching prior to exercise would loosen up our muscles and help prevent injuries; however, recent research has proven otherwise. It is now generally accepted that doing static stretches prior to a workout will be likely to make you slower and weaker during your exercise sessions and might actually *increase* your risk for injury.[1] Your best bet would be to do some active, sport-specific movements beforehand to adequately prepare your muscles for work. Then, you can focus on stretching *after* your workout, when your muscles are warm and much more elastic. So, for example, if you're going out for a jog, you could simply warm up with a fast-paced walk prior to starting, and then add in some basic stretches at the end. If you're interested in viewing some stretching videos, check out www.anytimehealth.com.

In order to make flexibility exercises a consistent part of your training regimen, you need to plan for it. A lot of people have a tendency to skip or scrimp on stretching. To avoid this, make sure to reserve the last 10 minutes of your session for stretching, and try not to let your schedule get in the way. After all, you wouldn't normally cut your lifting or cardio sessions short, would you?

YOUR 21-DAY NUTRITION AND FITNESS PLAN

This book is chock-full of information, but after discovering the how and the why, at the end of the day you still have to *do*. That's where this 21-day nutrition and fitness plan comes into play. Keep in mind, this program is designed to get beginners, both male and female, started off on the right foot. We provided everything you need to eat and exercise well for the next 21 days. You certainly don't need to follow this program word for word, but it will simplify things for you as you make the transition toward a healthier lifestyle. Then, after you've completed the program, you can either continue it or look for additional resources that can provide further guidance (www.anytimehealth.com would be a great place to start). If you have trouble sticking to it, go back and reread Part II, on changing behavior. Change can suck, as we all know, but Rebecca's advice in that section of the book will help you to persevere.

Before we send you on your way, there are a few things you should keep in mind from both the nutrition and the fitness perspectives.

NUTRITION

- The meal plan is based on a 2,000-calorie diet, but your calorie needs may be different. If that's the case, be sure to add or subtract foods as needed.
- If you want to substitute certain foods or beverages according to your likes and dislikes, please do. Just make sure that the food you substitute into the meal plan has a similar nutritional profile. For example, replacing a chicken breast with pork tenderloin is fine, but substituting a brownie for a banana is not. If you want to see the nutritional profile for a given food, use the diet tracker on www.anytimehealth.com.
- You'll notice that we made every effort to ensure that sodium was kept relatively low and that fiber was kept relatively high in the meal plan. Traditionally, Americans consume far too much sodium and take in very little fiber, so making these two simple dietary changes can go a long way toward better health.
- If your schedule doesn't allow you to eat five meals per day as our plan suggests, don't worry about it. Simply move those calories to another meal. In the end, a good meal plan must be flexible enough to accommodate even the busiest of schedules.

FITNESS

- The fitness plan represents *exercise*, but remember, you should still try to incorporate as much *physical activity* as you can into the rest of your day. This means taking walks, playing with your kids, and spending less time in front of the TV and computer.

- For the strength-training exercises, find a weight you can do no more than twelve to fifteen times, and use that as the starting point for your first set. Then, challenge yourself by increasing the weight by 5 to 10 pounds for the second set. The goal is to complete each set to failure.
- If you're unsure of how to do a particular strength-training exercise, check out the exercise videos on www.anytimehealth.com. You'll find both introductory and demonstration videos that will highlight the muscles being worked and the proper form, along with tips to keep in mind when you're performing the movements.
- Feel free to substitute strength-training exercises into your workout if there are some that you're unable to perform. You'll find plenty of options available for each muscle group on the Web site mentioned above. The key is to try to maintain muscular balance with the exercises you choose.
- If you find 20 or 30 minutes of steady-state cardiovascular exercise too difficult, that's fine. Start with whatever is most comfortable for you, and then gradually increase your duration each week. The focus should be on finding something challenging for you and your current fitness level. Walking, biking, jogging, rowing, and the elliptical machine are all great options.
- The fitness plan is laid out in an easy-to-follow format, but if your schedule gets in the way, just be sure to maintain at least one rest day between strength-training sessions. And don't be concerned about combining cardio and strength training on the same day if that works better for you.

- Finally, as with any new program, be sure to check with your doctor or health-care provider to make sure you're good to go.

There's no better time to start transforming your life than right now. Let's do it!

21-DAY MEAL PLAN

DAY 1

MONDAY
Calories: 1,913
Fat: 16.5%
Carbs: 57.1%
Protein: 26.3%
Sodium: 1,080 mg
Fiber: 51 g

BREAKFAST
1 cup black coffee
2 cups toasted oats cereal with 1 cup skim milk, and ½ cup
    strawberries

MORNING SNACK
15 whole wheat crackers with 2 tablespoons peanut butter

LUNCH
1 8-inch whole wheat tortilla with 4 ounces grilled chicken
    with ½ cup black beans, ½ cup brown rice, ¼ cup corn,
    ¼ cup tomatoes, and ¼ cup red onions
½ cup baby carrots

AFTERNOON SNACK
1 hardboiled egg
½ cup raspberries

DINNER
6 ounces roasted turkey breast, 1 cup mashed sweet
    potatoes, and 1½ cups green beans (cooked in olive oil)

Add 2 tablespoons ketchup for an additional 30 calories

Or add 3 tablespoons brown gravy for an additional 65 calories

DAY 1 FITNESS PLAN

MONDAY

Warm-up

5 minutes

Resistance

Seated shoulder press

Biceps curls

Triceps press machine

High row

Seated chest press

Floor crunches

Dumbbell side bends

Superman

Seated leg extension machine

Seated leg curl

REPEAT CIRCUIT FOR A TOTAL OF TWO SETS

Flexibility

Back and shoulder stretch

Overhead stretch

Calf stretch

Butterfly stretch

Hamstring stretch

DAY 2

TUESDAY
Calories: 1,988
Fat: 21.8%
Carbs: 51.2%
Protein: 27.0%
Sodium: 1,907 mg
Fiber: 47 g

BREAKFAST
1 cup fat-free skim milk
1 slice toasted whole wheat bread
2 egg whites scrambled
2 tablespoons salsa

MORNING SNACK
6 ounces plain yogurt with ½ cup blueberries
¼ cup dry-roasted, unsalted almonds

LUNCH
4 ounces sliced turkey breast, 2 slices tomato, ¼ cup spinach,
   and 1 slice cheddar cheese on an 8-inch whole wheat
   tortilla with 1 tablespoon light mayo and 1 tablespoon
   fat-free honey mustard
1 cup cantaloupe

AFTERNOON SNACK
1 cup low-fat cottage cheese
9 cherry tomatoes

DINNER
1 cup whole wheat spaghetti and 6 ounces soy balls
   (meatless "meatballs") with 2/3 cup marinara sauce (Soy

balls are made of mainly soy protein and chickpea flour.
They can be found at your local health-food stores)

6 large strawberries

1 cup steamed broccoli

EVENING SNACK

3 cups air-popped white popcorn

DAY 2 FITNESS PLAN

TUESDAY

Warm-up
   5 minutes

Cardio
   20 minutes

Cool-down
   5 minutes

Flexibility
   Butterfly stretch
   Hamstring stretch
   Calf stretch

DAY 3

WEDNESDAY
Calories: 2,050
Fat: 23.6%
Carbs: 51.8%
Protein: 24.6%
Sodium: 1,660 mg
Fiber: 47 g

BREAKFAST
1 egg omelet with ½ cup mushrooms, ¼ cup spinach, ¼ cup peppers, ⅛ cup onions, and 1 ounce cheddar cheese
1 cup black coffee

MORNING SNACK
1 medium banana
⅓ cup almonds
8 ounces skim milk

LUNCH
5 ounces shredded chicken on 2 slices whole wheat bread with 2 slices tomato, 1 ounce mozzarella cheese, and 1 tablespoon basil
½ cup strawberries

AFTERNOON SNACK
8 ounces skim milk
½ cup broccoli
½ cup cauliflower
2 tablespoons fat-free ranch dressing

DINNER

6 ounces beef stroganoff with 1¼ cup whole wheat pasta,
  1 cup portabella mushrooms
1 cup steamed asparagus

EVENING SNACK

½ cup strawberries, ½ cup raspberries with ½ cup plain
  yogurt
8 ounces 100% orange juice

DAY 3 FITNESS PLAN

WEDNESDAY

Warm-up
  5 minutes

Resistance
  Lateral raises
  Hammer curls
  Dumbbell kickbacks
  Lat pull-downs
  Bench press
  Rope crunches
  Side plank
  Superman
  Angle leg press
  Bosu tilts
  Repeat circuit for a total of two sets

Flexibility
  Back/oblique stretch
  Triceps stretch
  Chest stretch
  Inner thigh stretch
  Hamstring stretch

DAY 4

THURSDAY
Calories: 1,935
Fat: 22.2%
Carbs: 52.6%
Protein: 25.2%
Sodium: 1,450 mg
Fiber: 44 g

BREAKFAST
1½ cups oatmeal with ½ cup blueberries and 1 cup skim milk
1 slice whole wheat toast with 1 tablespoon unsalted butter

MORNING SNACK
⅓ cup mixed nuts (dry roasted, unsalted)
6 ounces 100% orange juice (100% juice, with pulp) (or reduced sugar)

LUNCH
6 ounces grilled salmon on 2 cups spinach salad with ¼ cup mandarin oranges, 1 tablespoon chopped pecans, and 2 tablespoons raspberry vinaigrette

AFTERNOON SNACK
1 cup baby carrots
1 cup sugar snap peas
3 tablespoons hummus

DINNER
one 8-inch whole wheat tortilla, 2 ounces mozzarella cheese, ⅓ cup green peppers, ⅓ cup spinach, ⅓ cup mushrooms, and 1 tablespoon reduced-fat sour cream
1 cup skim milk

DAY 4 FITNESS PLAN

THURSDAY

Warm-up
   5 minutes

Cardio
   20 minutes

Cool-down
   5 minutes

Flexibility
   Quadriceps stretch
   Hamstring stretch
   Calf stretch

DAY 5

FRIDAY
Calories: 1,910
Fat: 26.3%
Carbs: 47.4%
Protein: 26.3%
Sodium: 1600 mg
Fiber: 43 g

BREAKFAST
1 scrambled whole egg and 1 scrambled egg white with
    ¼ cup green peppers and ¼ cup mushrooms
1 plum

MORNING SNACK
1 large apple
2 tablespoons peanut butter

LUNCH
2 cups spinach with 4 ounces roasted turkey, ¼ cup red bell
    pepper, ½ cup cucumber, 1 tablespoon sunflower seeds,
    and 2 tablespoons low-fat Italian dressing
½ cup sugar snap peas, ½ cup celery
2 tablespoons garlic hummus
1 apricot

AFTERNOON SNACK
⅓ cup mixed nuts
¼ cup dried cranberries

DINNER
one 5-ounce grilled chicken breast
1 cup brown rice

1 cup green beans
½ cup blueberries

EVENING SNACK
1 slice angel food cake with ½ cup blackberries

DAY 5 FITNESS PLAN

FRIDAY

Warm-up
  5 minutes

Resistance
  Pec Deck rear shoulder machine
  Biceps curl machine
  Cable triceps push-downs
  Bent-over row
  Seated cable fly
  Reverse plank
  Torso rotations
  Lunges
  Deadlift
  Standing calf raises
  REPEAT CIRCUIT FOR A TOTAL OF TWO SETS

Flexibility
  Cat stretch
  Glute stretch
  Quadriceps stretch
  Hip stretch
  Chest stretch

DAY 6

SATURDAY
Calories: 1,961
Fat: 26.4%
Carbs: 51.5%
Protein: 22.1%
Sodium: 1,885 mg
Fiber: 45 g

BREAKFAST
1 cup low-fat vanilla yogurt with ¼ cup raspberries and
   ¼ cup granola
1 banana
1 cup black coffee

MORNING SNACK
1 medium orange
1 light string cheese stick

LUNCH
3 ounces ham on 2 slices whole wheat bread with 1 ounce
   low-sodium cheddar cheese, ½ cup spinach, and ¼ cup
   green pepper
1 cup of reduced-sodium tomato soup

AFTERNOON SNACK
¼ cup raisins
1 cup skim milk

DINNER
4 ounces tofu on 1 cup spaghetti squash with ¼ cup light
   Alfredo sauce (packaged) and 1 cup broccoli

EVENING SNACK

8 ounces 100% cranberry juice (reduced-sugar)

½ cup trail mix (unsalted)

DAY 6 FITNESS PLAN

SATURDAY

Warm-up

5 minutes

Cardio

20 minutes

Cool-down

5 minutes

Flexibility

Glute stretch

Hamstring stretch

Inner thigh stretch

SUNDAY
Calories: 1,917
Fat: 19.6%
Carbs: 54.5%
Protein: 26.0%
Sodium: 1,587 mg
Fiber: 44 g

BREAKFAST
1 cup oat bran cereal with ¾ cup skim milk and ¼ cup dried
  cherries
1 slice cinnamon raisin toast with 2 teaspoons Smart
  Balance

MORNING SNACK
1 cup low-fat plain yogurt with ¼ cup raspberries and
  ¼ cup blackberries
8 ounces skim milk

LUNCH
4 ounces grilled chicken on a whole wheat bun with
  1 ounce swiss cheese, 2 slices tomato, and 1 tablespoon
  low-fat mayo
2 cups mixed greens salad with ½ cup tomatoes, ½ cup
  carrots, ½ cup cucumber, and 1 tablespoon low-sodium
  Italian dressing

AFTERNOON SNACK
1 tablespoon peanut butter and 1 tablespoon jelly on 1 slice
  whole wheat bread

DINNER

Stir fry with 5 ounces beef over 1 cup brown rice and 1 cup
   mixed vegetables (red pepper, onion, mushrooms)

DAY 7 FITNESS PLAN

SUNDAY

Rest

DAY 8

MONDAY

Calories: 1,990

Fat: 24.0%

Carbs: 50.2%

Protein: 25.8%

Sodium: 1,993 mg

Fiber: 39 g

BREAKFAST

2 slices whole wheat cinnamon French toast and
2 tablespoons fruit spread

1 cup skim milk

MORNING SNACK

6 ounces low-fat yogurt and ¼ cup granola

LUNCH

6-ounce veggie burger on 1 whole wheat bun with ¼ cup
lettuce, 2 slices tomato, 1 teaspoon mustard, and
2 teaspoons ketchup

1 medium banana

AFTERNOON SNACK

1 ounce string cheese

⅓ cup dry unsalted almonds

DINNER

8 ounces grilled ahi tuna on 2 cups arugula salad with
½ cup roasted red peppers, ¼ cup red onions, ¼ cup
edamame, and 2 tablespoons balsamic vinaigrette

1 cup low-sodium vegetable soup

8 ounces skim milk

DAY 8 FITNESS PLAN

MONDAY

Warm-up
 5 minutes

Resistance
 Dumbbell front raises
 Cable biceps curls
 Overhead triceps extensions
 Cable row
 Dumbbell incline press
 Abdominal machine
 Oblique crunches
 Hip abduction machine
 Squats (bodyweight)
 Prone leg curl
 REPEAT CIRCUIT FOR A TOTAL OF TWO SETS

Flexibility
 Buttocks stretch
 Shoulder stretch
 Overhead stretch
 Trunk stretch
 Forearm stretch

DAY 9

TUESDAY
Calories: 2,011
Fat: 19.7%
Carbs: 54.5%
Protein: 25.8%
Sodium: 2,125 mg
Fiber: 44 g

BREAKFAST
1 whole wheat cinnamon raisin bagel with 2 tablespoons
   peanut butter
8 ounces 100% orange juice, low-sugar

MORNING SNACK
2 cups watermelon

LUNCH
1 cup low-sodium split pea with ham soup
1 kiwi fruit

AFTERNOON SNACK
1 large apple
¼ cup unsalted peanuts

DINNER
6 ounces spicy grilled chicken and 2 cups bell peppers, red
   onions, carrots, and broccoli
2 cups mixed greens with 2 tablespoons balsamic
   vinaigrette
2/3 cup chickpeas
8 ounces skim milk

DAY 9 FITNESS PLAN

TUESDAY

Warm-up
　5 minutes

Cardio
　20 minutes

Cool-down
　5 minutes

Flexibility
　Butterfly stretch
　Hamstring stretch
　Calf stretch

DAY 10

WEDNESDAY
Calories: 1,978
Fat: 22.4%
Carbs: 50.4%
Protein: 27.3%
Sodium: 1,501 mg
Fiber: 43 g

BREAKFAST
1½ cups mixed berries with 6 ounces low-fat yogurt
12 almonds

MORNING SNACK
15 baked tortilla chips with ½ cup refried beans and
    1 ounce low-fat cheddar cheese

LUNCH
10-inch whole wheat tortilla with 4 ounces sliced turkey
    breast, 1 slice swiss cheese, ¼ cup spinach, 1 slice tomato,
    ½ tablespoon light mayonnaise, and ¼ tablespoon honey
    mustard
8 ounces skim milk

AFTERNOON SNACK
12 pretzels

DINNER
6-ounce grilled salmon filet
1¼ cups cooked summer squash
1 cup whole-grain pasta

EVENING SNACK

½ cup light frozen yogurt

DAY 10 FITNESS PLAN

WEDNESDAY

Warm-up

5 minutes

Resistance

Seated cable shoulder press

Concentration curls

Single-arm reverse push-downs

Isolateral front lat pull-downs

Bench push-ups

Abdominal crunch bench

Cable reverse axe chop

Reverse bridge (with abduction)

Seated leg-press machine

Straight-leg deadlift

REPEAT CIRCUIT FOR A TOTAL OF TWO SETS

Flexibility

Back and shoulder stretch

Calf stretch

Butterfly stretch

Hamstring stretch

Back/oblique stretch

DAY 11

THURSDAY
Calories: 1,950
Fat: 23.4%
Carbs: 54.1%
Protein: 22.6%
Sodium: 1,773 mg
Fiber: 54 g

BREAKFAST
1 breakfast burrito: 2 eggs, 1 cup mixed vegetables, and
　1 ounce cheddar cheese on whole wheat tortilla
8 ounces 100% orange juice

MORNING SNACK
1 ounce toasted pita chips with ⅓ cup roasted red pepper
　hummus
1 large apple

LUNCH
5 ounces grilled eggplant and 5 ounces tofu (soft, silken) on
　1 whole wheat bun
1 large pear
6 ounces plain low-fat yogurt

AFTERNOON SNACK
1 ounce string cheese
1 cup strawberries

DINNER
2 slices whole wheat bread with 1 Boca burger, 1 slice
　cheddar cheese, 2 slices avocado, 2 slices tomato, and
　¼ cup lettuce

8 ounces skim milk

1 cup baby carrots

DAY 11 FITNESS PLAN

THURSDAY

Warm-up

   5 minutes

Cardio

   20 minutes

Cool-down

   5 minutes

Flexibility

   Quadriceps stretch

   Hamstring stretch

   Calf stretch

DAY 12

FRIDAY
Calories: 1,997
Fat: 16.4%
Carbs: 57.5%
Protein: 26.2%
Sodium: 1,264 mg
Fiber: 48 g

BREAKFAST
1 bran muffin (150 calories)
2 tablespoons apple butter
1 cup fresh blueberries
6 ounces black coffee

MORNING SNACK
1 cup plain yogurt with ¾ cup strawberries and
2 tablespoons raisins

LUNCH
4 ounces grilled chicken breast, ½ cup green peppers,
3 tablespoons sunflower seeds, and 1 cup corn salsa over
2 cups spinach
1 large peach

AFTERNOON SNACK
2 cups watermelon

DINNER
8 ounces skim milk
6 ounces roasted turkey breast with ¾ cup succotash and
¾ cup sweet potatoes
1 cup steamed broccoli

DAY 12 FITNESS PLAN

FRIDAY

Warm-up

 5 minutes

Resistance

 Cable rear shoulder fly

 Cable crossovers

 High pulley biceps curls

 Triceps extensions (dumbbell)

 Cable single-arm row

 Resistance-band chest press

 Crunches with medicine ball

 Dumbbell side bends

 Smith machine lunges

 Cable leg curls

 REPEAT CIRCUIT FOR A TOTAL OF TWO SETS

Flexibility

 Overhead stretch

 Forearm stretch

 Chest stretch

 Buttocks stretch

 Triceps stretch

 Trunk and back stretch

DAY 13

SATURDAY
Calories: 1,949
Fat: 25.5%
Carbs: 52.0%
Protein: 22.6%
Sodium: 2,350 mg
Fiber: 41 g

BREAKFAST
2 scrambled egg whites
1 pancake with 1½ cups strawberries, raspberries, and
blackberries

MORNING SNACK
6 ounces low-sugar pomegranate juice
6 ounces low-fat yogurt and 1 banana

LUNCH
5 ounces grilled chicken on a whole wheat bun with 1
ounce swiss cheese, 2 slices tomato, and 1 tablespoon
low-fat mayo
2 cups mixed greens salad with ⅓ cup tomatoes, ⅓ cup
carrots, ⅓ cup cucumber, and 2 tablespoons low-sodium
Italian dressing

AFTERNOON SNACK
2 tablespoons peanut butter and 2 tablespoons jelly on
2 slices whole wheat bread

DINNER
1 medium piece of vegetable lasagna and tomato sauce
(homemade or packaged)

½ cup steamed spinach

4 ounces mixed fruit

DAY 13 FITNESS PLAN

SATURDAY

Warm-up

   5 minutes

Cardio

   20 minutes

Cool-down

   5 minutes

Flexibility

   Glute stretch

   Hamstring stretch

   Inner thigh stretch

DAY 14

SUNDAY
Calories: 1,951
Fat: 23.5%
Carbs: 49.0%
Protein: 27.5%
Sodium: 1,661 mg
Fiber: 36 g

BREAKFAST
6 ounces 100% orange juice, low-sugar
2 egg white omelet with ⅛ cup onions, ⅛ cup red peppers,
⅛ cup mushrooms, ¼ cup spinach and ⅛ cup cheddar
cheese
1 whole wheat English muffin with 1 tablespoon Smart
Balance

MORNING SNACK
1 cup plain yogurt with ½ cup blueberries and ¼ cup
granola

LUNCH
3 ounces sliced turkey on 2 slices whole wheat bread with
1 ounce low sodium cheddar cheese and 1 tablespoon
Dijon mustard
1 cup of reduced-sodium tomato soup
8 ounces skim milk

AFTERNOON SNACK
1 cup skim milk blended with 1 medium banana and 1 cup
strawberries

DINNER

6 ounces oven-roasted halibut with 1 cup couscous and
   1 cup steamed asparagus

2 cups mixed greens salad with ⅛ cup tomatoes, ⅛ cup
   carrots, ⅛ cup cucumber, and 1 tablespoon low-sodium
   Italian dressing

DAY 14 FITNESS PLAN

SUNDAY

Rest

DAY 15

MONDAY

Calories: 1,960

Fat: 22.4%

Carbs: 48.1%

Protein: 29.4%

Sodium: 995 mg

Fiber: 35 g

BREAKFAST

8 ounces 100% cranberry juice

1 packet cinnamon instant oatmeal with 1 medium sliced apple (for the oatmeal)

MORNING SNACK

1½ cups low-sodium tomato soup

LUNCH

1 whole wheat bun with 6-ounce tuna filet, 2 tablespoons avocado, 2 slices tomato, ¼ cup spinach, and 1 teaspoon mustard

AFTERNOON SNACK

8 ounces skim milk

10 whole wheat crackers with 2 tablespoons peanut butter

DINNER

5 ounces roasted turkey breast with 1 cup mashed sweet potatoes, and 1 cup green beans

8 ounces skim milk

DAY 15 FITNESS PLAN

MONDAY

Warm-up

   5 minutes

Resistance

   Stability-ball shoulder press

   Alternating dumbbell curls

   Seated rope triceps extensions

   Straight-arm lat pull-down

   Stability-ball chest press

   Plank

   Torso rotations

   Walking lunges

   Bosu tilts

   Glute push

   REPEAT CIRCUIT FOR A TOTAL OF TWO SETS

Flexibility

   Cat stretch

   Overhead stretch

   Calf stretch

   Butterfly stretch

   Hamstring stretch

DAY 16

TUESDAY
Calories: 2,023
Fat: 34.6%
Carbs: 38.9%
Protein: 26.5%
Sodium: 1,736 mg
Fiber: 28 g

BREAKFAST
1 cup black coffee
1 cup plain yogurt with ½ cup strawberries
1 slice whole wheat toast with 1 tablespoon unsalted butter

MORNING SNACK
8 ounces skim milk
⅓ cup unsalted almonds
⅓ cup dried cranberries

LUNCH
5 ounces grilled salmon on 2 cups spring mix with ¼ cup
    red onion, ¼ cup carrots, ¼ cup cucumber, and
    2 tablespoons balsamic vinaigrette
1 cup low-sodium chunky vegetable soup

AFTERNOON SNACK
¼ cup unsalted cashews
⅓ cup blueberries

DINNER
6 ounces lean beef over 1 cup brown rice with ½ cup
    mushrooms and ½ cup onions

DAY 16 FITNESS PLAN

TUESDAY

Warm-up
  5 minutes

Cardio
  30 minutes

Cool-down
  5 minutes

Flexibility
  Butterfly stretch
  Hamstring stretch
  Calf stretch

DAY 17

WEDNESDAY
Calories: 1,961
Fat: 33.7%
Carbs: 41.8%
Protein: 24.4%
Sodium: 1,984 mg
Fiber: 44 g

BREAKFAST
6 ounces 100% orange juice
1 cup plain yogurt with ½ cup raspberries, ½ cup
    blackberries, and ¼ cup granola

MORNING SNACK
1 ounce toasted pita chips with ⅓ cup roasted red pepper
    hummus

LUNCH
2 slices whole wheat bread with 5 ounces grilled chicken,
    1 ounce cheddar cheese, 1 teaspoon honey Dijon
    mustard, and 2 slices avocado
1 cup baby carrots

AFTERNOON SNACK
½ grapefruit
8 ounces skim milk

DINNER
shrimp scampi made with 20 small shrimp, 1 cup whole
    wheat pasta, 1 tablespoon extra-virgin olive oil, and
    1 clove garlic
¾ cup spinach

EVENING SNACK

1 slice angel food cake with ¾ cup sliced strawberries and
½ tablespoon slivered almonds

DAY 17 FITNESS PLAN

WEDNESDAY

Warm-up
5 minutes

Resistance
Modified rear shoulder raises
Barbell curls
Bench dips
Barbell shrugs
Dumbbell fly
Stability-ball crunches
Back extensions
Stability-ball leg extensions
Reverse lunges
Seated calf raises
REPEAT CIRCUIT FOR A TOTAL OF TWO SETS

Stretching
Back/oblique stretch
Triceps stretch
Chest stretch
Inner thigh stretch
Hamstring stretch

DAY 18

THURSDAY
Calories: 1,977
Fat: 13.4%
Carbs: 69.6%
Protein: 17.0%
Sodium: 2,427 mg
Fiber: 49 g

BREAKFAST
1 cup black coffee
1 pancake with ¼ cup raspberries, ¼ cup blueberries, ¼ cup
 strawberries, and 1 tablespoon honey

MORNING SNACK
1 cup baby carrots with 2 tablespoons fat-free ranch
 dressing
1 banana
8 ounces skim milk

LUNCH
1½ cups low-sodium bean and ham soup
1 cup mixed greens salad with ¼ cup fresh red bell pepper,
 ¼ cup cucumber, ⅛ cup red onion, and 2 tablespoons fat-
 free French dressing
6 ounces plain yogurt with ½ cup pineapple and ⅓ cup
 granola

AFTERNOON SNACK
⅓ cup bean dip with 15 baked tortilla chips

DINNER

6 ounces beef and vegetable goulash over 1 cup brown rice

1 cup steamed broccoli

8 ounces skim milk

DAY 18 FITNESS PLAN

THURSDAY

Warm-up

5 minutes

Cardio

30 minutes

Cool-down

5 minutes

Flexibility

Quadriceps stretch

Hamstring stretch

Calf stretch

DAY 19

FRIDAY

Calories: 1,951

Fat: 26.6%

Carbs: 47.0%

Protein: 26.3%

Sodium: 2,283 mg

Fiber: 33g

BREAKFAST

8 ounces 100% orange juice (low-sugar)

2 cups toasted oats cereal with 1 cup skim milk, ½ cup
   pitted cherries, and ¼ cup chopped almonds

1 cup low-fat plain yogurt with ¼ cup raspberries

LUNCH

Reuben sandwich: 6 ounces sliced turkey, ⅛ cup
   sauerkraut, and 1 tablespoon avocado on 2 slices rye
   bread

2 cups arugula salad with ¼ cup tomatoes and 1 tablespoon
   balsamic vinaigrette

AFTERNOON SNACK

½ cup edamame

8 ounces skim milk

DINNER

5 ounces meatloaf with 1 cup mashed potatoes, 1 cup mixed
   vegetables (carrots, broccoli, and peas), and ¼ cup gravy

EVENING SNACK

1 apricot

DAY 19 FITNESS PLAN

FRIDAY

Warm-up

    5 minutes

Resistance

    Medicine-ball front raises

    Speed-ball curls

    Stability-ball dumbbell triceps extensions

    Cable lat pull-downs

    Modified push-ups

    Bicycle crunches

    Side plank with abduction

    Sumo squat

    Hip extensions

    Kneeling hip abduction

    REPEAT CIRCUIT FOR A TOTAL OF TWO SETS

Flexibility

    Cat stretch

    Glute stretch

    Quadriceps stretch

    Hip stretch

    Chest stretch

DAY 20

SATURDAY
Calories: 2,069
Fat: 32.4%
Carbs: 37.8%
Protein: 29.9%
Sodium: 2,312 mg
Fiber: 41 g

BREAKFAST
2 slices of whole wheat toast with 2 tablespoons peanut
    butter and 1 banana
1 cup skim milk

MORNING SNACK
1 cup carrot sticks and 1 cup celery sticks
⅓ cup unsalted almonds

LUNCH
one 8-inch whole wheat tortilla with 6 ounces spicy grilled
    chicken, 1 ounce swiss cheese, 2 tablespoons salsa, ¼ cup
    shredded lettuce, and 1 ounce avocado
1 small apple

AFTERNOON SNACK
1 ounce string cheese

DINNER
8 ounces grilled ahi tuna on 2 cups arugula salad with
    ½ cup roasted red peppers and ¼ cup red onions
1 cup steamed asparagus

EVENING SNACK

1 large peach

DAY 20 FITNESS PLAN

SATURDAY

Warm-up
   5 minutes

Cardio
   30 minutes

Cool-down
   5 minutes

Flexibility
   Glute stretch
   Hamstring stretch
   Inner thigh stretch

DAY 21

SUNDAY
Calories: 2,035
Fat: 24.2%
Carbs: 52.2%
Protein: 23.5%
Sodium: 630 mg
Fiber: 39 g

BREAKFAST
1 cup cinnamon oatmeal with 1 large apple
1 cup skim milk

MORNING SNACK
1 cup grapes
1 cup plain yogurt
¼ cup granola

LUNCH
1½ cups hearty minestrone soup with ½ cup brown rice and
    ½ cup black beans

AFTERNOON SNACK
1 ounce low-sodium trail mix
8 ounces skim milk

DINNER
6 ounces oven-roasted halibut with 1 cup couscous and
    1½ cups steamed asparagus

EVENING SNACK
¼ cup almonds
4 dark chocolate Hershey kisses

DAY 21 FITNESS PLAN

SUNDAY

Rest

ACKNOWLEDGMENTS

To our hardworking team members at Anytime Fitness corporate: Work is our play, and you inspire us with endless energy, collaboration, passion, empathy and humor. The journey continues . . .

To the quiet, clever, and creative Tara Dosh: Without your connections, this book might not have happened, or it would never have happened this fast. And your talents in editing, story development, PR, and writing have been a valuable resource throughout this project.

To David Tripp: Eighteen months to publish a book? Yeah . . . right! Thank you for listening to our foolishness and championing the cause.

To the formidable editing and project management duo of Renee Sedliar and Christine E. Marra: You kept a rapidly moving train from veering off the track. Your steadfast guidance, support, and expertise enabled three first-time authors to navigate the complex world of publishing.

Lissa Warren: PR people don't suck, but we appreciate your helping us spread the word that working out does!

FROM CHUCK: Rebecca and Brian, thank you for embracing this task without hesitation and agreeing to the uncommonly short timeline. Carpe diem.

To Marc Conklin for helping me shape this book and providing critical, honest feedback and creative suggestions. Your influence goes beyond *WOS*, and you've made the brand of Anytime Fitness better. That's a cool gift.

To Dave Mortensen, my business partner and heart-first friend: Success doesn't happen alone, and the ride continues, with laughter, competitions, teamwork, and shared family moments.

To Shannon, Conik, Delaney, Ella, and Charlie: I start and end each day with you. I am a lucky guy. Love you.

FROM BRIAN: To my fellow colleagues, Debbie Pias and Samantha Donegan, for helping to craft a practical 21-day plan that's really doable.

To Becky, Megan, Lily, and Chase: If family defines happiness, then I'm the happiest guy in the world. Couldn't imagine life without you!

FROM REBECCA: To Chuck Runyon, for your intelligent, savvy leadership and your integrity. You lead from the "skinny branches," making dreams a reality. Brian Zehetner, thanks for your knowledge and commitment to excellence.

To Tara Dosh, for your insightful commentary and kind, intelligent approach to the editing process. Renee Sedliar and Christine Marra, thank you for your patience, creative editing, and belief in *WOS*.

To Mark, a beloved peacemaker. I think about you every day and will never forget you. To my clients, for your courage to face your pain and your commitment to emotional health. You are the best teachers I know.

To my brother, Christopher, the bravest person I know. My mother, Jacqueline, taught me to live authentically and creatively.

To Horowitz, Beethoven, and The Little Prince, my muse.

To Chris, for your kindness and unconditional love.

NOTES

PART 1: WORKING OUT SUCKS, BUT . . .

THE MAGIC PILL

1. See, for example, Daniel M. Landers, "The Influence of Exercise on Mental Health," *President's Council on Physical Fitness and Sports Research Digest* 2, no. 12 (1997), available at www.fitness.gov/mentalhealth.htm.

MUGGING YOURSELF

1. For more information on topics in this chapter, see Anytime Fitness, "The Existence Close and Overcoming the Money Objection," Anytime Fitness Community blog, 2011, www.anytimefitness.com/en-us/franchisee/community/blog/2011/3/7/The_Existence_Close_and_Overcoming_the_Money_Objection.

"AS LONG AS IT'S HEALTHY"

1. For general information on starting a healthy lifestyle, see President's Council on Fitness, Sports and Nutrition, Web page, www.fitness.gov; U.S. Department of Health and Human Services, "Quick Guide to Healthy Living," www.healthierus.gov; U.S. Department of Health and Human Services, "2008 Physical Activity Guidelines for Americans," last updated September 14, 2011, www.health.gov/paguidelines; and President's Council on Fitness, Sports and Nutrition, "President's Challenge," ww.presidentschallenge.org.

SEAT BELTS, CIGARETTES, AND CHILDHOOD OBESITY

1. For more on the role of parents in childhood obesity, see Lindsey Tanner, "Really Obese Kids May Need Foster Care, Two

Experts Argue," *(Minneapolis) Star Tribune*, July 13, 2011, www.
startribune.com/lifestyle/wellness/125460753.html; Chris Wool-
ston, "Placing Obese Children in Foster Homes a Controversial
Proposition," *Los Angeles Times*, July 14, 2011, http://articles.
latimes.com/2011/jul/14/news/la-heb-child-obesity-foster-care
-20110714; and Michelle L. Brandt, "Obese Parents Increase Kids'
Risk of Being Overweight," *Stanford Report*, Stanford University,
July 21, 2004, http://news.stanford.edu/news/2004/july21/med
-obesity-721.html.

iDEATH

1. For more information on the problems of inactivity, see Centers for Disease Control and Prevention, "Leading Causes of Death,"
final 2007 data, www.cdc.gov/nchs/fastats/lcod.htm; Centers for
Disease Control and Prevention, "February Is American Heart
Month," January 31, 2011, www.cdc.gov/features/heartmonth/; and
President's Council on Fitness, Sports and Nutrition, Web page,
www.fitness.gov.

DOES GARFIELD HAVE THE FAT GENE?

1. See, for example, Jeff Strickler, "Exercise and the Couch-
Potato Pooch," *(Minnesota) Star Tribune*, March 29, 2011, www.
startribune.com/lifestyle/118855594.html; and Ernest Ward Jr., "Pet
Obesity Continues to Grow in US," March 9, 2010, Association for
Pet Obesity, www.petobesityprevention.com/pet-obesity-grow-in
-us/.

MONEY IS ALLERGIC TO FAT PEOPLE

1. For more information on poverty and obesity, see Sharon
Jayson, "Study: Beautiful People Cash In on Their Looks," *USA Today*, March 31, 2011, www.usatoday.com/money/perfi/basics/2011
-03-30-beauty30_ST_N.htm; and Eve Tahmincioglu, "Fat Chance:
It's Not Easy for Obese Workers," Careers on msnbc.com, 2011,
www.msnbc.msn.com/id/16755130/ns/business-personal_finance
/t/fat-chance-its-not-easy-obese-workers/.

I LOVE MILFS!

1. See, for example, Michelle L. Brandt, "Obese Parents Increase Kids' Risk of Being Overweight," *Stanford Report*, Stanford University, July 21, 2004, http://news.stanford.edu/news/2004/july21/med -obesity-721.html; President's Council on Fitness, Sports and Nutrition, Web page, www.fitness.gov; and U.S. Department of Health and Human Services, "Quick Guide to Healthy Living," www. healthierus.gov.

FOOD DOES NOT SUCK

1. For help on facing this war, see, for example, *Fooducate* Blog, "Our Fat Future," June 4, 2011, www.fooducate.com/blog/2011/06/ 04/our-fat-future-eye-opening-infographic/.

COOKING THE BOOKS

1. Lorien E. Urban et al., "Accuracy of Stated Energy Contents of Restaurant Foods," *Journal of the American Medical Association*, July 20, 2011. See also Daniela Hernandez, "What's on the Menu? More Calories Than Listed, Study Finds," *St. Paul Pioneer Press*, July 20, 2011, www.twincities.com/ci_18510389?IADID=Search -www.twincities.com.

(IT'S UP TO) YOU

1. David Brown, "Global Epidemic, 1 in 10 of World's Adults Are Diabetic," *Washington Post*, June 26, 2011.

2. "U.S. Adults Keep Getting Fatter," *Minneapolis Star Tribune*, July 7, 2011.

3. Ibid.

PART 2: CHANGING BEHAVIOR SUCKS, TOO, BUT ...

INTRODUCTION

1. Norman Doidge, *The Brain That Changes Itself: Stories of Personal Triumph from the Frontier of Brain Science* (New York: Penguin, 2007).

2. Stephen Covey, *The Seven Habits of Highly Effective People* (New York: Simon & Schuster, 1989).

BEGIN WITH THE END IN MIND (with thanks to Stephen Covey)

1. Maxwell Maltz and Bobbe Sommer, *Psycho-Cybernetics 2000* (Paramus, NJ: Prentice Hall, 2000).

2. Martha J. Farah, Lauren L. Weisberg, Mark Monheit, and Franck Peronnet, "Brain Activity Underlying Visual Imagery: Event-Related Potentials During Mental Image Generation," *Journal of Cognitive Neuroscience* 1 (1989): 302–316.

3. Norman Doidge, *The Brain That Changes Itself: Stories of Personal Triumph from the Frontier of Brain Science* (New York: Penguin, 2007).

MIND OVER MATTER

1. Daniel Amen, *Change Your Brain, Change Your Life: The Breakthrough Program for Conquering Anxiety, Depression, Obsessiveness, Anger, and Impulsiveness* (New York: Three Rivers Press, 2000).

2. Joseph LeDoux, *Synaptic Self: How Our Brains Become Who We Are* (New York: Penguin, 2002).

3. Phillippa Lally, Cornelia H. M. van Jaarsveld, Henry W. W. Potts, and Jane Wardle, "How Are Habits Formed: Modelling Habit Formation in the Real World," *European Journal of Social Psychology* 40, no. 6 (2010): 998–1009.

I WOULD KILL FOR CHOCOLATE!

1. Bruce Perry and Ronnie Pollard, "Homeostasis, Stress, Trauma, and Adaptation: A Neurodevelopmental View of Childhood Trauma," *Child and Adolescent Psychiatric Clinics of North America* 7, no. 1 (January 1998): 33–51.

2. Norman Doidge, *The Brain That Changes Itself: Stories of Personal Triumph from the Frontier of Brain Science* (New York: Penguin, 2007).

EVERY MOUNTAINEER STUMBLES: THE MYTH OF PERFECTION

1. Randy O. Frost, Patricia Marten, Cathleen Lahart, and Robin Rosenblate, "The Dimensions of Perfectionism," *Cognitive Therapy & Research* 14, no. 5 (1990): 449–468.

2. Ibid.

STRENGTH IN NUMBERS

1. Kerry Patterson, Joseph Grenny, David Maxfield, Ron McMillan, and Al Switzler, *Change Anything: The New Science of Personal Success* (New York: Business Plus, 2011).

2. Ibid.

PART 3: NUTRITION SUCKS, TOO, BUT . . .

THE CARB CRAZINESS

1. A. Welsh, A. J. Sharma, L. Grellinger, and M. B. Vos, "Consumption of Added Sugars Is Decreasing in the United States," *American Journal of Clinical Nutrition* 94, no. 3 (2011): 726–734, available at www.ncbi.nlm.nih.gov/pubmed/21753067.

2. Rachel K. Johnson et al., "Dietary Sugars Intake and Cardiovascular Health: A Scientific Statement from the American Heart Association," *Circulation* 120 (2009): 1011–1020.

3. S. M. Moeller, S. A. Fryhofer, A. J. Osbahr III, and C. B. Robinowitz, "The Effects of High-Fructose Corn Syrup," *Journal of the American College of Nutrition* 28, no. 6 (2009): 619–626.

GO FIBER OR GO HOME

1. Jane Higdon, "Fiber," Linus Pauling Institute, Oregon State University, December 2005, available at http://lpi.oregonstate.edu/infocenter/phytochemicals/fiber/.

2. Panel on Macronutrients, Panel on the Definition of Dietary Fiber, Subcommittee on Upper Reference Levels of Nutrients, Subcommittee on Interpretation and Uses of Dietary Reference Intakes, and the Standing Committee on the Scientific Evaluation

of Dietary Reference Intakes, *Dietary Reference Intakes for Energy, Carbohydrate, Fiber, Fat, Fatty Acids, Cholesterol, Protein, and Amino Acids* (Washington, DC: Food and Nutrition Board, Institute of Medicine of the National Academies, 2009), 389.

3. U.S. Department of Health and Human Services, Food and Drug Administration, Center for Food Safety and Applied Nutrition, Office of Nutrition, Labeling and Dietary Supplements, *Food Labeling Guide* (Washington, DC: FDA, October 2009).

PROTEIN: THE PERFECT BUILDING MATERIAL

1. U.S. Department of Agriculture, Agricultural Research Service, USDA Nutrient Data Laboratory, *USDA National Nutrient Database for Standard Reference*, Release 23, 2010.

SIMPLIFYING THE FATS ISN'T SO SIMPLE

1. A. P. Simopoulos, "The Importance of the Ratio of Omega-6/Omega-3 Essential Fatty Acids," *Biomedicine and Pharmacotherapy* 56 (2002): 365–379.

THE 411 ON H$_2$O

1. H. Valtin, "'Drink At Least Eight Glasses of Water per Day.' Really? Is There Scientific Evidence for '8 × 8'?" *American Journal of Physiology, Regulatory, Integrative and Comparative Physiology* 283 (2002): R993–1004.

2. Panel on Dietary Reference Intakes for Electrolytes and Water, Standing Committee on the Scientific Evaluation of Dietary Reference Intakes, *Dietary Reference Intakes for Water, Potassium, Sodium, Chloride, and Sulfate,* (Washington, DC: National Academies Press, 2005), 145–147.

3. E. A. Dennis et al., "Water Consumption Increases Weight Loss During a Hypocaloric Diet Intervention in Middle-Aged and Older Adults," *Obesity* 18 (2010): 300–307.

4. From U.S. Department of Agriculture, Agricultural Research Service, USDA Nutrient Data Laboratory, "USDA National Nutrient Database for Standard Reference," Release 23, 2010).

5. Mark Bittman, "Bad Food? Tax It, and Subsidize Vegetables," *New York Times*, July 23, 2011.

TO SUPPLEMENT OR NOT, THAT IS THE QUESTION

1. Council for Responsible Nutrition, "Dietary Supplements: Safe, Beneficial and Regulated," Council for Responsible Nutrition, Washington, DC, revised March 14, 2011, www.crnusa.org/CRN RegQandA.html.

2. Centers for Disease Control and Prevention, "Dietary Supplement Use Among U.S. Adults Has Increased Since NHANES III (1988–1994)," NCHS Data Brief no. 61, April 2011, www.cdc.gov/nchs/data/databriefs/db61.htm.

3. M. A. Tarnopolsky, "Effect of Caffeine on the Neuromuscular System—Potential as an Ergogenic Aid," *Applied Physiology, Nutrition, and Metabolism* 33 (2008): 1284–1289.

A "WEIGHTY" ISSUE

1. U.S. Department of Health and Human Services, Weight-Control Information Network, "Overweight and Obesity Statistics," updated February 2010, http://win.niddk.nih.gov/statistics/.

2. T. S. Church et al., "Trends over 5 Decades in U.S. Occupation-Related Physical Activity and Their Associations with Obesity," *PLoS One* 6 (2011): e19657.

3. "Weight Cycling: National Task Force on the Prevention and Treatment of Obesity," *Journal of the American Medical Association* 272 (October 19, 1994): 1196–1202.

4. National Weight Control Registry, "NWCR Facts," National Weight Control Registry, Providence, RI, www.nwcr.ws/Research/default.htm, accessed July 14, 2011.

GIMME THE NUTRITIONAL GAME PLAN

1. U.S. Department of Health and Human Services and U.S. Department of Agriculture, "Dietary Guidelines for Americans, 2010," January 31, 2011, www.health.gov/dietaryguidelines/.

2. Nanci Hellmich, "Many Americans Clueless of How Many Calories They Do or Should Eat," *USA Today*, July 7, 2010.

PART 4: FITNESS SUCKS, TOO, BUT . . .

MOVING IS NEAT

1. J. A. Levine et al., "Interindividual Variation in Posture Allocation: Possible Role in Human Obesity," *Science* 307 (2005): 584–586.

THE CARDIO PRESCRIPTION

1. E. Garber et al., "Quantity and Quality of Exercise for Developing and Maintaining Cardiorespiratory, Musculoskeletal, and Neuromotor Fitness in Apparently Healthy Adults: Guidance for Prescribing Exercise," *Medicine & Science in Sports & Exercise* 43 (2011): 1334–1359.

2. David M. Buchner et al., *2008 Physical Activity Guidelines for Americans* (Washington, DC: U.S. Department of Health and Human Services, 2008), vii.

IS STRENGTH THE NEW CARDIO?

1. C. E. Garber et al., "Quantity and Quality of Exercise for Developing and Maintaining Cardiorespiratory, Musculoskeletal, and Neuromotor Fitness in Apparently Healthy Adults: Guidance for Prescribing Exercise," *Medicine & Science in Sports & Exercise* 43 (2011): 1334–1359.

2. J. LaForgia, R. T. Withers, and C. J. Gore, "Effects of Exercise Intensity and Duration on the Excess Post-Exercise Oxygen Consumption," *Journal of Sports Sciences* 24 (2006): 1247–1264.

STRETCH MUCH?

1. See, for example, C. E. Garber et al., "Quantity and Quality of Exercise for Developing and Maintaining Cardiorespiratory, Musculoskeletal, and Neuromotor Fitness in Apparently Healthy Adults: Guidance for Prescribing Exercise," *Medicine & Science in Sports & Exercise* 43 (2011): 1334–1359.

INDEX

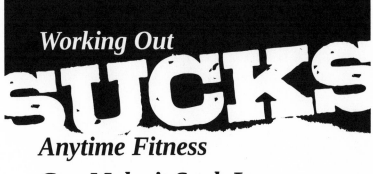

Working Out SUCKS

Anytime Fitness
Can Make it Suck Less

**Free
30-Day
Pass**

ANYTIME FITNESS is the best place for fitness 24/7. Friendly, affordable, inspiring, and fun! Bring this ad to your local Anytime Fitness today. Find a location near you at **AnytimeFitness.com**.

**Free
Premuim
12-Month
Pass**

ANYTIME HEALTH is your online resource for living well. Plan meals, track workouts, get expert advice, and connect with friends! Click "Sign up Now" on **AnytimeHealth.com** – select "Premium" and enter code WOS2012.

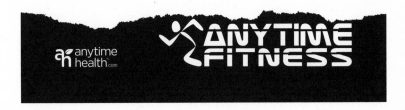

anytime health.com

ANYTIME FITNESS